P9-CMT-660

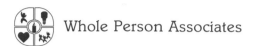
Whole Person Associates

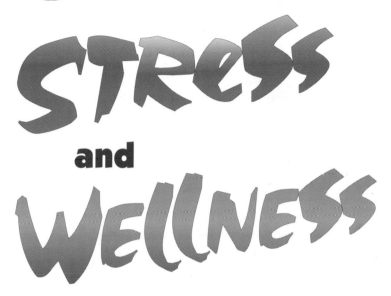

# STRESS and WELLNESS

## Reference Guide

A Comprehensive Index to the
Chalktalks, Processes, and Activities
in the Whole Person
Structured Exercises Series

Nancy Loving Tubesing, EdD

Copyright © 1995 by Whole Person Associates Inc

All rights reserved. Except for short excerpts for review purposes, no part of this book may be reproduced or transmitted in any form by any means, electronic or mechanical, without permission in writing from the publisher.

Whole Person Associates
210 West Michigan
Duluth MN 55802-1908
218-727-0500

ISBN 1-57025-080-4

Printed in the United States of America by Versa Press
10 9 8 7 6 5 4 3 2 1

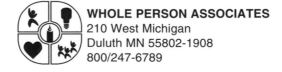

**WHOLE PERSON ASSOCIATES**
210 West Michigan
Duluth MN 55802-1908
800/247-6789

# ▦ INTRODUCTION

This *Reference Guide* was developed at the request of trainers, teachers, and group leaders in the field who regularly use ideas and activities from the Whole Person *Structured Exercises in Stress Management* and *Wellness Promotion* series in their teaching, consulting, or clinical practice. This handy index provides a key to the 382 teaching designs in those volumes, organized in several different ways to help you locate content and processes to meet your needs and fit your audience.

## ▦ Visual Index                                                  p. 1

As a starting point, see the *Visual Index,* p. 1–33. This comprehensive guide shows every exercise, grouped by section, with an easy-to-read chart indicating volume, page number, minimum/maximum time, effective group size, materials needed (worksheets, handouts, A-V resources, scripts, other materials), workplace appropriateness, and processes (introductions, chalktalks, demonstrations, relaxation routines, group activities, small group sharing, large group discussion). The *Visual Index* also outlines the level of self-disclosure for participants, the level of expertise/preparation for the leader, and favorite exercises of the series editors.

## ▦ Exercise Descriptions                                          p. 118

If you would like to know more about any of the exercises in the *Visual Index,* or if you are looking for learning experiences to meet specific goals and objectives, you will find complete descriptions of each exercise, along with goals and time frame, in the *Exercise Descriptions* section. This is the place to scan the Table of Contents for each volume in the series.

## ▦ Annotated Indexes                                             p. 34

If you are looking for specific content material or thematic group experiences, check out the *Annotated Indexes* which briefly summarize the content and process of lecturettes (called *chalktalks*), demonstrations, mental and physical energizers, and relaxation routines in the ten volumes of the series, with appropriate page numbers for easy reference.

## ▓ Winning Combinations                                    p. 62

The *Winning Combinations* section includes thirty stress and wellness presentation/workshop outlines, ranging from 45 minutes to a full day to several weekly sessions—all using combinations of structured exercises from one or more volumes in the series. If you're looking for fresh ideas, or a new approach to these timely topics, use these outlines as a springboard for your own creativity.

## ▓ Editors' Choice                                         p. 78

The editors of these series have chosen several exercises in each volume as favorites. After more than twenty years of teaching about stress and wellness we know that these are truly gems—so we gave them our four-star rating. When you need something in a hurry that is guaranteed to work well with nearly any group, trust these four-star *Editors' Choices*.

## ▓ Especially for the Workplace                           p. 89

Every volume in the *Stress* and *Wellness* series includes group processes that are especially effective in the workplace. If you would like to address issues unique to the job setting, or use techniques that work especially well with work teams, explore the exercises suggested in the *Especially for the Workplace* index.

## ▓ Tips for Trainers                                       p. 98

Don't miss the *Tips for Trainers* section, a mini continuing professional education seminar, featuring great advice for planning and conducting presentations and workshops using the *Structured Exercises* series. Whether you are a novice health educator or a senior consultant, you'll find practical tips here that will enhance your effectiveness.

## ▓ Contributors                                    p. 169

The *Structured Exercises in Stress Management* and *Wellness Promotion* series are grounded in the philosophy of the Big Circle—experienced teachers and presenters sharing the best of their knowledge with others in the field, so that more people can be encouraged to develop and maintain healthy, satisfying lifestyles. The *Contributors* section highlights those seasoned veterans who have so generously shared their expertise in these volumes.

## ▓ Title Index                                     p. 179

Finally, if you are looking for a specific exercise you remember by name, try the *Title Index*. Once you begin browsing this intriguing list, you may get caught up in reading it all the way through—just for the fun of it. There's a goldmine of good ideas in the titles alone.

## ▓ Note on Abbreviations

Throughout this *Reference Guide*, books in the series are referred to by acronyms: S1 for *Structured Exercises in Stress Management, Volume 1*, (S2, S3, S4, S5 for others in the *Stress* series) and W1 for *Structured Exercises in Wellness Promotion, Volume 1*, (W2, W3, W4, W5 for others in the *Wellness* series.

Specific exercises are noted with the exercise number following the volume number (eg, S1.1a, W5.161).

# ◼ CONTENTS

## 4 EDITORS' CHOICE ................................. 78

Editors' favorite exercises from the ten volumes.

## 5 ESPECIALLY FOR THE WORKPLACE ................................. 89

Structured exercises in stress and wellness that are particularly appropriate for work environments.

## 6 TIPS FOR TRAINERS ................................. 98

Complete *Tips for Trainers* sections from each volume of the series.

# 7 EXERCISE DESCRIPTIONS ................................. 118

A brief overview of each exercise listed by volume. Includes time frame
and specific goals.

# 8 CONTRIBUTORS ..................................... 169

A mini-biography of contributors to the ten volumes of *Structured
Exercises in Stress Management* and *Wellness Promotion.*

# TITLE INDEX .......................................... 179

# WHOLE PERSON PRODUCTS........................... 184

# 1
# Visual Index to Exercises

These short (5–20 minutes) and lively exercises are designed to introduce people to each other and to the subject. *Stress* and *Wellness* series.

These exercises help people explore the symptoms, sources, and dynamics of stress and examine the impact of stress in their lives. Adaptable to various settings, audiences, and time frames. *Stress* series.

Participants evaluate their strengths and weaknesses and identify skills for future development, as they explore overall strategies for dealing with the stress of life. *Stress* series.

Each volume in the *Stress* series focuses on four or five practical coping skills in more depth.

Moderate-length assessments (30–60 minutes) and major theme developers (60–90 minutes) explore the issue of wellness from the whole person perspective. Rather than focusing merely on the physical, these processes help people examine their total lifestyle. *Wellness* series.

These exercises (10–60 minutes) promote personal responsibility for well-being. Participants examine their self-care patterns and explore specific self-care strategies in different life dimensions: physical (diet, relaxation, fitness); mental; relational; spiritual; and lifestyle well-being. *Wellness* series.

These exercises help participants draw together their insights and determine actions they wish to take on their own behalf. Some also provide rituals that bring closure to the group process. *Stress* and *Wellness* series.

These quick energizers are designed to perk up the group whenever fatigue sets in. Sprinkle them throughout your program to illustrate skills or concepts. Try one for a change of pace—everyone's juices (including yours!) will be flowing again in 5–10 minutes. *Stress* and *Wellness* series.

**Volume**
S1, S2, S3, S4, S5: *Structured Exercises in Stress Management, Volumes 1–5.*
W1, W2, W3, W4, W5: *Structured Exercises in Wellness Promotion, Volumes 1–5.*

**Exercise #**
Exercises in each series (*Stress* and *Wellness*) are numbered consecutively from 1 to 180. Some exercises are actually collections of similar, but unique processes (identified as a, b, c).

**Page #**
Refers to the location of the exercise in its volume. Please note: occasionally there is a one-page difference between the location of an exercise in the looseleaf and softcover editions.

**Min/Max Time**
Minimum (bare bones, sharing in 2s or 3s).
Maximum (including all options, sharing in groups of 4–6).

**Group Size**
U = Unlimited
I = Works well with individuals
< # = Best for group smaller than designated number.
> # = Best for group larger than the designated number.

**Blackboard**
A ■ in this column indicates the need for a chalkboard, newsprint easel, or overhead projector.

**A-V Needed**
A ✓ in this column indicates the need for A-V equipment (projector/TV-VCR, portable sound system, cassette/CD player, etc). Check the original exercise for specifics.

**Materials**
A ✂ in this column means that the exercise requires additional materials ranging from art supplies to reference books to Tinkertoys. Check the original exercise for specifics.

**Worksheets**
A ✎ marks exercises that include essential worksheets for participant reflection, assessment, or planning. For more information on obtaining full-size worksheet masters, see p. 184.

**Handouts**
A ❑ marks exercises that include handouts for participants (eg, song lyrics, charts, instructions, etc). Most handouts are included in the worksheet master packets, or you can easily substitute other formats for presenting the information.

**Worksite**
Exercises with a ◆ in this column deal with workplace stress/wellness issues or are especially effective for use in job settings or work teams.
For a complete listing of worksite-appropriate exercises, see the *Especially for the Workplace Index,* beginning on p. 89.

**Favorites**
Exercises marked with a ☆ in this column are the special favorites of the series editors.
For more information on these four-star exercises, see the complete list in the *Editors' Choice* section, beginning on p. 78.

**Introductions**
Exercises marked with a ◆ in this column include some kind of get-acquainted process.

**Chalktalk**
A ● in this column indicates that the trainer is expected to present information to participants in a lecturette. Basic content is included in the chalktalk points outlined in the exercise, but every trainer/leader will want to adapt the presentation to your own approach and personalize it with examples.
For content of specific chalktalks, see the *Chalktalk Index,* p. 35.

**Demo**  A ➤ in this column points out an exercise that includes a demonstration. These range from *in vivo* stress arousal experiences to modeling a stretch routine or relaxation technique. For more information, consult the complete list of demonstrations in all ten volumes, p. 45.

**Relaxation**  Exercises marked with a ◆ in this column incorporate some form of physical and/or mental relaxation. A complete list of all routines, with brief descriptions, begins on p. 58.

**Script**  The symbol 🎙 appears in this column when the exercise includes a script to be read by the trainer. Scripts range from guided imagery to parables.

**Activity**  Any exercise marked with a ◆ in this column includes at least one large group activity, such as a mixer, game, movement experience, creative venture, or other process that involves activity. For more details, see the specific exercise description and accompanying goals in the *Exercise Descriptions,* p. 118.

**Small groups**  Nearly all of the 382 exercises in these ten volumes incorporate some form of interpersonal interaction. Exercises marked with a ❖ include significant use of small groups (2–8 people) for sharing and discussion.

**Large group**  Exercises with a ✳ in this column include at least a brief time for discussion and input from the entire group.

**Disclosure**  The Whole Person *Structured Exercises* are based on the conviction that learning and motivation are powerfully enhanced when people share their insights and plans for change with others in small groups. However, different levels of disclosure may be appropriate with different audiences and in different settings.

To determine the self-disclosure level of a particular exercise, compare the number in this column to the key below.

Blank = No significant self-disclosure.

    ❶ = Brief/low-level sharing in response to open-ended questions of nonsensitive nature; individual chooses how much to disclose.

    ❷ = Personal sharing in response to direct questions about somewhat sensitive issues. Opportunity for disclosure of current strengths/problems. Feedback/affirmation.

    ❸ = Opportunity for deeper disclosure about potentially painful subjects. Pointed questions/assessment.

**Trainer Prep**  As you skim through the list of exercises, take note of this column which reveals the amount of preparation required on the part of the trainer—including gathering of necessary materials as well as the experience level of the leader.

Blank = No prep time needed, ready to go as is.

    ❶ = Easy, but needs materials or preparation.

    ❷ = Some preparation needed; content/process suitable to most trainers.

    ❸ = Longer/more complicated exercise; requires extensive preparation and/or sophisticated judgement by trainer.

| VOLUME | EXERCISE # | PAGE # | EXERCISE TITLE | MIN TIME TO MAX TIME | GROUP SIZE | BLACKBOARD | A-V NEEDED | MATERIALS | WORKSHEETS | HANDOUTS |
|---|---|---|---|---|---|---|---|---|---|---|
| | | | **ICEBREAKERS** | | | | | | | |
| S1 | 1a | 1 | Life Windows | 10–30 | U | | | ✂ | | |
| S1 | 1b | 2 | Stress Collage | 10–30 | U | | | ✂ | | |
| S1 | 1c | 3 | Rummage Sale | 10–30 | <20 | | | ✂ | | |
| S1 | 2 | 5 | Relaxation Bingo | 10–20 | 15–50 | | | | ✏ | |
| S1 | 3 | 7 | Clear the Deck! | 10–15 | U | | | | | |
| S1 | 4 | 10 | Two–Minute Drill | 10–15 | U, I | | | ✂ | | |
| S1 | 5 | 13 | Stress Breaks | 15 | U | | | ✂ | | |
| S1 | 6 | 15 | Personal Stressors and Copers | 20–30 | U | ■ | | | | |
| | | | | | | | | | | |
| S2 | 37a | 1 | Alphabet Copers | 10–20 | U | | | | | |
| S2 | 37b | 2 | Personal/Professional | 10–20 | U | | | | | |
| S2 | 37c | 2 | Wave the Magic Wand | 10–20 | U | | | | | |
| S2 | 38 | 5 | Turtle, Hare, or Racehorse? | 20–30 | 15–40 | | | ✂ | | |
| S2 | 39 | 9 | Four Quadrant Questions | 25–30 | U | | | ✂ | | |
| S2 | 40 | 12 | Life Event Bingo | 10–30 | >15 | | | | ✏ | |
| S2 | 41 | 14 | Exclusive Interview | 25–30 | U | | | | | ❑ |
| | | | | | | | | | | |
| S3 | 73a | 1 | Models | 10–20 | U | | | | | |
| S3 | 73b | 2 | Under Fire | 10–20 | U | | | ✂ | | |
| S3 | 74 | 4 | Agenda Consensus | 15 | <30 | ■ | | ✂ | | |
| S3 | 75 | 6 | Marauders | 20–30 | U | ■ | | | | |
| S3 | 76 | 10 | Pandora's Box | 10–15 | 6–12 | | | ✂ | | |
| S3 | 77 | 12 | Traveling Trios | 10–15 | >16 | | | | | |
| S3 | 78 | 14 | Going to Jerusalem | 10–20 | <20 | | | | | |
| | | | | | | | | | | |
| S4 | 109a | 1 | Coping Choreography | 10–20 | U | | | | | |
| S4 | 109b | 2 | Barometer | 10–20 | U | | | | | |
| S4 | 110 | 3 | Family Yarns | 10–20 | U | | | ✂ | | |
| S4 | 111 | 5 | Quips and Quotes | 20–30 | U | | | ✂ | | ❑ |

KEY on page 2

| CATEGORY | EXERCISE # | WORKSITE | FAVORITES | INTRODUCTIONS | CHALKTALK | DEMO | RELAXATION | SCRIPT | ACTIVITY | SMALL GROUPS | LARGE GROUP | DISCLOSURE | TRAINER PREP |
|---|---|---|---|---|---|---|---|---|---|---|---|---|---|
| **Stress 1** | | | | | | | | | | | | | |
| | 1a | | ☆ | ◆ | | | | | | ⁘ | | ❷ | ❶ |
| | 1b | | | ◆ | | | | | ◆ | | ✳ | | ❷ |
| | 1c | | | ◆ | | | | | | | ✳ | ❶ | ❶ |
| | 2 | | | ◆ | | | | | ◆ | ⁘ | ✳ | | ❶ |
| | 3 | | ☆ | | | | ◆ | 99 | | | ✳ | | ❶ |
| | 4 | | | ◆ | | | | 99 | | ⁘ | | ❷ | ❷ |
| | 5 | | | ◆ | | | ◆ | | ◆ | ⁘ | ✳ | | ❶ |
| | 6 | | | ◆ | | | | | | ⁘ | ✳ | ❷ | |
| **Stress 2** | | | | | | | | | | | | | |
| | 37a | ◆ | | ◆ | | | | | | | ✳ | | |
| | 37b | ◆ | | ◆ | | | | | | | ✳ | ❶ | |
| | 37c | | | ◆ | | | | | | | ✳ | ❷ | |
| | 38 | | | ◆ | ● | | | | ◆ | ⁘ | ✳ | ❶ | ❶ |
| | 39 | | ☆ | ◆ | ● | | | | | ⁘ | ✳ | ❷ | ❶ |
| | 40 | | | ◆ | | | | | ◆ | ⁘ | ✳ | ❷ | ❶ |
| | 41 | | | ◆ | | | | | | ⁘ | ✳ | | |
| **Stress 3** | | | | | | | | | | | | | |
| | 73a | | | ◆ | | | | | | | ✳ | ❶ | |
| | 73b | | | ◆ | | ➤ | | | ◆ | ⁘ | ✳ | | ❷ |
| | 74 | ◆ | | | ● | | | | | | ✳ | ❶ | ❶ |
| | 75 | | | | ● | ➤ | | | ◆ | ⁘ | ✳ | ❷ | ❶ |
| | 76 | | | | | | | | | | ✳ | ❶ | ❶ |
| | 77 | | | ◆ | | | | | ◆ | ⁘ | ✳ | ❶ | ❶ |
| | 78 | | | ◆ | | | | | | | ✳ | ❶ | |
| **Stress 4** | | | | | | | | | | | | | |
| | 109a | | | ◆ | ● | | | | | | ✳ | ❶ | |
| | 109b | | | ◆ | | | | | | | ✳ | ❶ | |
| | 110 | | | ◆ | | | | | | | ✳ | ❷ | ❶ |
| | 111 | | ☆ | ◆ | | | | | | ⁘ | ✳ | ❶ | |

KEY on page 2

©1995 Whole Person Press 210 W Michigan Duluth MN 55802 (800) 247-6789

| VOLUME | EXERCISE # | PAGE # | EXERCISE TITLE | MIN TIME TO MAX TIME | GROUP SIZE | BLACKBOARD | A-V NEEDED | MATERIALS | WORKSHEETS | HANDOUTS |
|---|---|---|---|---|---|---|---|---|---|---|
| | | | **ICEBREAKERS** | | | | | | | |
| S4 | 112 | 10 | Count Five | 10–15 | >20 | | | ✂ | | |
| S4 | 113 | 12 | Dear Me | 10–15 | U | | | | ✎ | |
| S4 | 114 | 14 | Wanted Posters | 15–20 | U | | | ✂ | ✎ | |
| | | | | | | | | | | |
| S5 | 145a | 1 | Symbols | 5–15 | U | | | ✂ | | |
| S5 | 145b | 2 | Birthday Party | 5–15 | U | | | | | |
| S5 | 146 | 4 | Badge of My Profession | 15–20 | U | | | ✂ | ✎ | |
| S5 | 147 | 7 | Nametag Questions | 15–20 | U | | | ✂ | | |
| S5 | 148 | 10 | One-Minute Autobiographies | 10–20 | 8–16 | ■ | | ✂ | | |
| S5 | 149 | 12 | Pace Setters | 5–10 | U | | | | | |
| S5 | 150 | 14 | Ton of Bricks | 15–20 | U | | | ✂ | | |
| | | | | | | | | | | |
| W1 | 1a | 1 | Analogies | 5–10 | U | | | | | |
| W1 | 1b | 2 | Affirmations | 5–10 | U | | | ✂ | | |
| W1 | 1c | 2 | Wellness Goals/Health Concerns | 5–10 | U | | | ✂ | | |
| W1 | 1d | 3 | Jingles | 5–10 | U | | | | | |
| W1 | 2 | 5 | Two-Minute Mill | 10–15 | U | | | | | |
| W1 | 3 | 8 | Human Health/Illness Continuum | 10–20 | >20 | | | | | |
| W1 | 4 | 11 | Beautiful People Pin-Up Contest | 10–20 | U | ■ | | ✂ | | |
| W1 | 5 | 14 | Ten Qualities of the Super Well | 25–30 | U | ■ | | | ✎ | |
| | | | | | | | | | | |
| W2 | 37a | 1 | Roundup | 10–15 | U | | | | | |
| W2 | 37b | 2 | Differences | 10–15 | U | | | | | |
| W2 | 37c | 3 | Pocket or Purse | 10–15 | U | | | | | |
| W2 | 38 | 4 | "Quality" Circles | 10–15 | U | | | ✂ | | |
| W2 | 39 | 6 | Attention to Tension | 15–20 | U | | | | | |
| W2 | 40 | 8 | Silent Auction | 20–30 | 8–24 | | | ✂ | ✎ | |
| W2 | 41 | 14 | Vitality Score | 5–10 | U | | | | | |

KEY on page 2

| CATEGORY | EXERCISE # | WORKSITE | FAVORITES | INTRODUCTIONS | CHALKTALK | DEMO | RELAXATION | SCRIPT | ACTIVITY | SMALL GROUPS | LARGE GROUP | DISCLOSURE | TRAINER PREP |
|---|---|---|---|---|---|---|---|---|---|---|---|---|---|
| **Stress 4** | | | | | | | | | | | | | |
| | 112 | | | ◆ | | ➤ | | | ◆ | ✣ | ✳ | | ❶ |
| | 113 | | ☆ | ◆ | | | | | | | ✳ | ❶ | ❶ |
| | 114 | | | | | | | | | ✣ | | ❷ | ❶ |
| **Stress 5** | | | | | | | | | | | | | |
| | 145a | | | ◆ | | | | | ◆ | ✣ | | ❶ | ❶ |
| | 145b | | | ◆ | | | | | | ✣ | ✳ | | |
| | 146 | ◆ | | ◆ | | | | | ◆ | ✣ | | ❷ | ❶ |
| | 147 | | | ◆ | | | | | ◆ | ✣ | ✳ | | ❷ |
| | 148 | | ☆ | ◆ | | ➤ | | | | ✣ | | ❶ | ❶ |
| | 149 | ◆ | | ◆ | ● | ➤ | | | | | | ❶ | |
| | 150 | | | ◆ | ● | ➤ | | | | ✣ | | ❶ | ❶ |
| **Wellness 1** | | | | | | | | | | | | | |
| | 1a | ◆ | | ◆ | | | | | | | ✳ | | |
| | 1b | | | ◆ | | | | | | ✣ | | ❶ | |
| | 1c | ◆ | | ◆ | | | | | | ✣ | | ❶ | ❶ |
| | 1d | | | ◆ | | | | | | ✣ | | | |
| | 2 | ◆ | ☆ | ◆ | | ➤ | | | ◆ | ✣ | ✳ | ❶ | |
| | 3 | | | ◆ | | | | | ◆ | ✣ | ✳ | ❶ | ❶ |
| | 4 | | | ◆ | | | | | ◆ | | ✳ | | ❶ |
| | 5 | | | ◆ | | | | | | ✣ | ✳ | ❶ | ❶ |
| **Wellness 2** | | | | | | | | | | | | | |
| | 37a | | | ◆ | | | | | | | ✳ | ❶ | |
| | 37b | ◆ | | ◆ | | | | | | | ✳ | ❶ | |
| | 37c | | ☆ | ◆ | | | | | | | ✳ | ❶ | |
| | 38 | ◆ | | ◆ | | | | | | ✣ | | ❶ | ❶ |
| | 39 | | | ◆ | ● | | ◆ | | ◆ | ✣ | ✳ | ❶ | |
| | 40 | | | | ● | | | | ◆ | | ✳ | ❷ | ❷ |
| | 41 | | | | | | | | | ✣ | ✳ | ❶ | |

KEY on page 2

©1995  Whole Person Press 210 W Michigan Duluth MN 55802     (800) 247-6789

| VOLUME | EXERCISE # | PAGE # | EXERCISE TITLE | MIN TIME TO MAX TIME | GROUP SIZE | BLACKBOARD | A-V NEEDED | MATERIALS | WORKSHEETS | HANDOUTS |
|---|---|---|---|---|---|---|---|---|---|---|
| | | | **ICEBREAKERS** | | | | | | | |
| W3 | 73a | 1 | My Mother Says | 10–15 | U | | | | | |
| W3 | 73b | 2 | Sabotage and Self-Care | 10–15 | U | | | | | |
| W3 | 73c | 2 | Simon Says | 10–15 | U | | | | | |
| W3 | 74 | 4 | Saturday Night Live! | 20–30 | U | | | | | |
| W3 | 75 | 6 | Health-Oriented People Hunt | 15–20 | U | | | ✂ | ✎ | |
| W3 | 76 | 10 | Part of Me | 2–3 | U | | | | | |
| W3 | 77 | 12 | Getting to Know You | 20–30 | U | | | ✂ | | |
| W3 | 78 | 14 | Galloping Gourmet | 20–30 | U | | | ✂ | | |
| | | | | | | | | | | |
| W4 | 109a | 1 | An Apple a Day | 10–15 | U | | | ✂ | | |
| W4 | 109b | 2 | Hippocratic Humors | 10–15 | U | ■ | | | | |
| W4 | 109c | 3 | TP Tales | 10–15 | U | | | ✂ | | |
| W4 | 110 | 4 | Lost and Found | 10–15 | U | | | ✂ | | |
| W4 | 111 | 6 | Hearts at Risk | 10–15 | U | ■ | | | | |
| W4 | 112 | 8 | Magic Door | 10–15 | U, I | | | | | |
| W4 | 113 | 11 | Wheel of Fortune | 10–15 | U | | | | | ❑ |
| W4 | 114 | 14 | Wellness Emblem | 15–20 | U | | | | ✎ | |
| | | | | | | | | | | |
| W5 | 145a | 1 | Anchors Aweigh | 5–10 | U | | | | | |
| W5 | 145b | 2 | Imaginary Ball Toss | 5–10 | 8–10 | | | | | |
| W5 | 145c | 3 | I See Myself | 5–10 | U | ■ | | | | |
| W5 | 146 | 4 | Fact or Fiction | 10–15 | U | | | | ✎ | |
| W5 | 147 | 7 | Health Transcript | 15–20 | U | | | | ✎ | |
| W5 | 148 | 10 | Self-Esteem Pyramid | 15–20 | U | | | | | |
| W5 | 149 | 12 | TO DO Lists | 10–15 | U | | | | ✎ | |

KEY on page 2

| CATEGORY | EXERCISE # | WORKSITE | FAVORITES | INTRODUCTIONS | CHALKTALK | DEMO | RELAXATION | SCRIPT | ACTIVITY | SMALL GROUPS | LARGE GROUP | DISCLOSURE | TRAINER PREP |
|---|---|---|---|---|---|---|---|---|---|---|---|---|---|
| **Wellness 3** | | | | | | | | | | | | | |
| | 73a | | | ◆ | | | | | | | ✳ | ❶ | |
| | 73b | | | ◆ | | | ◆ | | | | ✳ | ❶ | |
| | 73c | | | ◆ | | | | | | | ✳ | | |
| | 74 | | | ◆ | | | | | ◆ | ✤ | ✳ | | |
| | 75 | | ☆ | ◆ | | | | | ◆ | | ✳ | ❶ | ❷ |
| | 76 | ◆ | | ◆ | | | | | | | ✳ | ❶ | ❷ |
| | 77 | | | ◆ | | | | | | ✤ | | ❶ | ❶ |
| | 78 | | | ◆ | | | | | | ✤ | | ❶ | ❷ |
| **Wellness 4** | | | | | | | | | | | | | |
| | 109a | | | ◆ | | | | | | ✤ | | ❶ | ❶ |
| | 109b | | | ◆ | ● | | | | | | ✳ | ❶ | |
| | 109c | ◆ | | ◆ | | | | | | | ✳ | ❶ | ❶ |
| | 110 | | | ◆ | | | | | | | ✳ | ❷ | ❶ |
| | 111 | ◆ | | ◆ | ● | | | | | ✤ | ✳ | | |
| | 112 | | | ◆ | | | ◆ | 99 | | | ✳ | | |
| | 113 | | ☆ | ◆ | | | | | ◆ | ✤ | | ❶ | ❶ |
| | 114 | | ☆ | ◆ | | | | | | ✤ | ✳ | ❷ | ❶ |
| **Wellness 5** | | | | | | | | | | | | | |
| | 145a | | | ◆ | | | | | | | ✳ | ❶ | |
| | 145b | | | ◆ | | | | | | | ✳ | ❶ | |
| | 145c | | | ◆ | | | | | | | ✳ | ❶ | |
| | 146 | ◆ | ☆ | ◆ | | | | | | ✤ | ✳ | ❶ | ❶ |
| | 147 | | | ◆ | | | | | | ✤ | ✳ | ❶ | ❶ |
| | 148 | | | ◆ | | | | | | ✤ | | ❷ | |
| | 149 | ◆ | | ◆ | ● | | | | | ✤ | ✳ | ❶ | ❶ |

KEY on page 2

©1995 Whole Person Press 210 W Michigan Duluth MN 55802     (800) 247-6789

| VOLUME | EXERCISE # | PAGE # | EXERCISE TITLE | MIN TIME TO MAX TIME | GROUP SIZE | BLACKBOARD | A-V NEEDED | MATERIALS | WORKSHEETS | HANDOUTS |
|---|---|---|---|---|---|---|---|---|---|---|
| | | | **STRESS ASSESSMENTS** | | | | | | | |
| S1 | 7 | 17 | Stress Symptom Inventory | 30–40 | U, I | | | | ✏ | |
| S1 | 8 | 22 | The Juggling Act | 40–60 | U | ■ | | | ✏ | |
| S1 | 9 | 28 | Stressful Occupations Contest | 35–45 | >20 | ■ | | ✂ | | |
| S1 | 10 | 32 | Stress Risk Factors | 10–20 | U, I | ■ | | | ✏ | |
| S1 | 11 | 37 | Lifetrap 1: Workaholism | 60–90 | U | | | | ✏ | |
| S2 | 42 | 17 | The Fourth Source of Stress | 45–60 | U | | | | ✏ | |
| S2 | 43 | 25 | Burnout Index | 10–15 | U, I | | | | ✏ | |
| S2 | 44 | 28 | Dragnet | 30–40 | U | | | | ✏ | |
| S2 | 45 | 32 | Back to the Drawing Board | 50–75 | U | | | ✂ | | |
| S2 | 46 | 36 | Lifetrap 2: Hooked on Helping | 60–90 | U | | | ✂ | ✏ | |
| S2 | 47 | 46 | Circuit Overload | 15–20 | U | ■ | | | ✏ | |
| S3 | 79 | 17 | Spice or Arsenic? | 20–30 | U | | | | ✏ | |
| S3 | 80 | 21 | On the Spot | 30–60 | U | | | ✂ | ✏ | ▯ |
| S3 | 81 | 26 | Drainers and Energizers | 10–25 | U | | | | ✏ | |
| S3 | 82 | 30 | Lifetrap 3: Sick of Change | 60–90 | U | ■ | | ✂ | ✏ | |
| S3 | 83 | 40 | Job Descriptions | 60 | 8–20 | | | ✂ | ✏ | |
| S3 | 84 | 44 | The Last Christmas Tree | 20–30 | 6–10 | | | | ✏ | |
| S4 | 115 | 17 | Stress Spider Web | 20–30 | 6–24 | ■ | | | ✏ | |
| S4 | 116 | 21 | Body Mapping | 30–45 | U | | | ✂ | | |
| S4 | 117 | 25 | On the Job Stress Grid | 25–40 | U | ■ | | | ✏ | |
| S4 | 118 | 33 | Stress Attitudes Survey | 20–30 | 12–30 | | | ✂ | | |
| S4 | 119 | 37 | Stress Sketch | 30–40 | U, I | | | ✂ | | |
| S4 | 120 | 41 | Lifetrap 4: Good Grief? | 60–90 | U | | | | ✏ | |
| S5 | 151 | 17 | The Hardiness Factor | 30–40 | U, I | | | ✂ | ✏ | |
| S5 | 152 | 22 | Lifetrap 5: Superwoman Syndrome | 60–90 | U | ■ | | ✂ | ✏ | |
| S5 | 153 | 34 | Pick Your Battles | 30 | U | | | | ✏ | |
| S5 | 154 | 38 | Stormy Passages | 20–30 | U | | | ✂ | ✏ | |
| S5 | 155 | 43 | Windows on Stress | 30–45 | U | ■ | | ✂ | ✏ | |

KEY on page 2

| CATEGORY | EXERCISE # | WORKSITE | FAVORITES | INTRODUCTIONS | CHALKTALK | DEMO | RELAXATION | SCRIPT | ACTIVITY | SMALL GROUPS | LARGE GROUP | DISCLOSURE | TRAINER PREP |
|---|---|---|---|---|---|---|---|---|---|---|---|---|---|
| Stress 1 | 7 | | ☆ | | | | | | | ✣ | ✳ | ❷ | ❶ |
| | 8 | ◆ | | | ● | | | | | ✣ | ✳ | ❷ | ❶ |
| | 9 | ◆ | | | ● | | | | ◆ | ✣ | ✳ | ❶ | ❶ |
| | 10 | | | | ● | | | | | | ✳ | ❶ | ❶ |
| | 11 | ◆ | | | ● | | | | ◆ | ✣ | ✳ | ❷ | ❸ |
| Stress 2 | 42 | | | | ● | | | | | ✣ | ✳ | ❷ | ❷ |
| | 43 | ◆ | | | ● | | | | | | ✳ | ❷ | ❶ |
| | 44 | | | | ● | | | | | ✣ | ✳ | ❷ | ❶ |
| | 45 | ◆ | ☆ | | ● | | | | ◆ | ✣ | ✳ | ❷ | ❶ |
| | 46 | ◆ | | ◆ | ● | | | | | ✣ | ✳ | ❷ | ❸ |
| | 47 | | ☆ | | ● | | | | | | ✳ | ❶ | ❶ |
| Stress 3 | 79 | | ☆ | ◆ | ● | | | | ◆ | ✣ | ✳ | ❷ | ❶ |
| | 80 | | | | ● | | | | | ✣ | ✳ | ❷ | ❷ |
| | 81 | | ☆ | | | | | | | | ✳ | ❶ | ❶ |
| | 82 | | | ◆ | ● | | | | | ✣ | ✳ | ❷ | ❸ |
| | 83 | ◆ | | | | | | | | ✣ | ✳ | ❶ | ❷ |
| | 84 | | | | | | ◆ | 99 | | | ✳ | ❸ | ❶ |
| Stress 4 | 115 | | | | | | | | | ✣ | ✳ | ❷ | ❶ |
| | 116 | | | | ● | ➤ | ◆ | | ◆ | ✣ | | ❷ | ❷ |
| | 117 | ◆ | | | ● | | | | | ✣ | ✳ | ❷ | ❷ |
| | 118 | | | | | | | | ◆ | ✣ | ✳ | ❶ | ❶ |
| | 119 | | ☆ | | | | | | ◆ | ✣ | ✳ | ❷ | ❷ |
| | 120 | | | | ● | | | | | ✣ | ✳ | ❸ | ❸ |
| Stress 5 | 151 | ◆ | | | ● | | | | ◆ | ✣ | ✳ | ❶ | ❷ |
| | 152 | ◆ | ☆ | | ● | | | | ◆ | ✣ | ✳ | ❷ | ❸ |
| | 153 | | | | ● | | | | | ✣ | ✳ | ❷ | ❶ |
| | 154 | | ☆ | | ● | | | 99 | | ✣ | ✳ | ❷ | ❶ |
| | 155 | | ☆ | | ● | | | | | ✣ | ✳ | ❷ | ❶ |

KEY on page 2

©1995 Whole Person Press 210 W Michigan Duluth MN 55802    (800) 247-6789

| VOLUME | EXERCISE # | PAGE # | EXERCISE TITLE | MIN TIME TO MAX TIME | GROUP SIZE | BLACKBOARD | A-V NEEDED | MATERIALS | WORKSHEETS | HANDOUTS |
|---|---|---|---|---|---|---|---|---|---|---|
| | | | **MANAGEMENT STRATEGIES** | | | | | | | |
| S1 | 12 | 49 | The AAAbc's of Stress Mgmt | 45–60 | U | ■ | | | ✎ | |
| S1 | 13 | 56 | Professional Self-Care | 60 | U | ■ | | | ✎ | |
| S1 | 14 | 63 | Coping Skills Assessment | 45–60 | U, I | | | | ✎ | |
| S1 | 15 | 68 | Skill Skits | 60 | >50 | ■ | | | | ☐ |
| S1 | 16 | 71 | Stress Buffer Shield | 20–30 | U, I | | | | ✎ | |
| | | | | | | | | | | |
| S2 | 48 | 49 | I've Got Rhythm | 15–20 | U, I | | | | ✎ | |
| S2 | 49 | 54 | PILEUP Copers | 60 | U, I | | | ✂ | | |
| S2 | 50 | 61 | Month of Fundays | 20–30 | U | | | | ✎ | |
| S2 | 51 | 64 | The Worry Stopper | 30–40 | U | | | | ✎ | |
| S2 | 52 | 70 | Consultants Unlimited | 30–45 | 10–30 | ■ | | ✂ | | |
| | | | | | | | | | | |
| S3 | 85 | 49 | Metaphors | 40–50 | U | | | ✂ | ✎ | |
| S3 | 86 | 54 | S.O.S. for Stress | 30–50 | U | | | ✂ | | |
| S3 | 87 | 59 | Stress Clusters Clinic | 40–60 | 18–24 | | | ✂ | ✎ | |
| S3 | 88 | 66 | Corporate Presentation | 20–30 | 30–60 | ■ | | ✂ | | |
| S3 | 89 | 68 | Imagine Success | 15–30 | U, I | | | | | |
| | | | | | | | | | | |
| S4 | 121 | 49 | A Good Stress Manager | 30–60 | 12–24 | | | ✂ | ✎ | ☐ |
| S4 | 122 | 56 | Obligation Overload | 45 | U | | | | | |
| S4 | 123 | 61 | Metaphors 2 | 20–30 | U | | | | ✎ | |
| S4 | 124 | 65 | 911 Emergency Plan | 20–30 | U, I | ■ | | ✂ | | |
| S4 | 125 | 68 | Rest in Peace | 15–20 | U, I | | | | ✎ | |
| | | | | | | | | | | |
| S5 | 156 | 49 | Managing Job Stress | 20–60 | U | | ✓ | | ✎ | |
| S5 | 157 | 51 | Questionable Copers | 30–40 | U | ■ | | | ✎ | |
| S5 | 158 | 55 | Silver Linings | 20–30 | U | | | ✂ | | |
| S5 | 159 | 59 | Stress Management Alphabet | 50–60 | U | ■ | | ✂ | ✎ | |
| S5 | 160 | 66 | Yesterday, Today, and Tomorrow | 20–30 | U | | | | ✎ | |

KEY on page 2

| CATEGORY | EXERCISE # | WORKSITE | FAVORITES | INTRODUCTIONS | CHALKTALK | DEMO | RELAXATION | SCRIPT | ACTIVITY | SMALL GROUPS | LARGE GROUP | DISCLOSURE | TRAINER PREP |
|---|---|---|---|---|---|---|---|---|---|---|---|---|---|
| **Stress 1** | | | | | | | | | | | | | |
| | 12 | | ☆ | | ● | ➤ | | | | ✛ | ✳ | | ❶ |
| | 13 | ◆ | | | | | | | | ✛ | ✳ | ❶ | ❶ |
| | 14 | | ☆ | | ● | | | | | | | | ❶ |
| | 15 | | | | | | | | ◆ | ✛ | | | ❶ |
| | 16 | | | | | | | | | ✛ | ✳ | | ❶ |
| **Stress 2** | | | | | | | | | | | | | |
| | 48 | | ☆ | | ● | ◆ | | | ◆ | | ✳ | | ❶ |
| | 49 | | | | ● | | | | ◆ | ✛ | ✳ | ❷ | ❷ |
| | 50 | | | | ● | | | | ◆ | | | | ❶ |
| | 51 | | ☆ | | ● | | | | ◆ | | ✳ | ❶ | ❶ |
| | 52 | ◆ | | | | | | | | | ✳ | | ❶ |
| **Stress 3** | | | | | | | | | | | | | |
| | 85 | | ☆ | | ● | | | | | ✛ | | ❶ | ❷ |
| | 86 | | ☆ | | ● | | | | | | ✳ | | ❶ |
| | 87 | | | | | | | | | ✛ | | | ❷ |
| | 88 | | | | | | | | | ✛ | | | ❶ |
| | 89 | | | | ● | | | 99 | | ✛ | | ❶ | ❶ |
| **Stress 4** | | | | | | | | | | | | | |
| | 121 | ◆ | | | ● | | | | ◆ | ✛ | ✳ | ❶ | ❷ |
| | 122 | ◆ | | | ● | | | | ◆ | ✛ | ✳ | ❷ | ❷ |
| | 123 | | ☆ | | ● | | | | | ✛ | ✳ | ❷ | ❸ |
| | 124 | | ☆ | | ● | | | | | | ✳ | | ❶ |
| | 125 | | | | ● | | | 99 | | ✛ | ✳ | ❶ | ❶ |
| **Stress 5** | | | | | | | | | | | | | |
| | 156 | ◆ | | ◆ | | | ◆ | | | ✛ | | ❶ | ❶ |
| | 157 | | | | ● | | | | | ✛ | ✳ | ❷ | ❶ |
| | 158 | | | | ● | | | | | | ✳ | ❷ | ❶ |
| | 159 | ◆ | | | ● | ➤ | ◆ | | ◆ | ✛ | | ❶ | ❷ |
| | 160 | | ☆ | ◆ | ● | | | | | ✛ | ✳ | ❶ | ❶ |

KEY on page 2

©1995  Whole Person Press 210 W Michigan Duluth MN 55802        (800) 247-6789

| VOLUME | EXERCISE # | PAGE # | EXERCISE TITLE | MIN TIME TO MAX TIME | GROUP SIZE | BLACKBOARD | A-V NEEDED | MATERIALS | WORKSHEETS | HANDOUTS |
|---|---|---|---|---|---|---|---|---|---|---|
| | | | **SKILL BUILDERS** | | | | | | | |
| S1 | 17 | 73 | Unwinding | 20–30 | U | | ✓ | | | |
| S1 | 18a | 78 | Goodbye | 2–5 | U | | | ✂ | | |
| S1 | 18b | 79 | The Allowing Attitude | 2–5 | U | | | | | |
| S1 | 18c | 80 | Slow Me Down Lord | 2–5 | U | | | | | |
| S1 | 19a | 82 | The Best Medicine | 5–10 | U | | | | | |
| S1 | 19b | 84 | Beloved Husband of Irma | 5–10 | U | | ✓ | | | |
| S1 | 19c | 84 | Flight of Fancy | 5–10 | U | | | | | |
| S1 | 20 | 86 | 5–4–3–2–1 Contact | 20–30 | >20 | | | ✂ | | |
| | | | | | | | | | | |
| S2 | 53 | 73 | Attitude Adjustment Hour | 25–35 | U | | | | | |
| S2 | 54 | 77 | Speak Up! | 40–45 | U | ■ | | | | |
| S2 | 55 | 81 | Affirmative Action Plan | 40–50 | U | ■ | | | ✎ | |
| S2 | 56 | 88 | Anchoring | 30 | U | | | | | |
| S2 | 57 | 92 | The ABC's of Time | 40–50 | U | | | | ✎ | |
| | | | | | | | | | | |
| S3 | 90 | 73 | Conflict Management | 60 | U | ■ | | | ✎ | |
| S3 | 91 | 80 | Eight-Minute Stress Break | 10 | U | | ✓ | ✂ | | |
| S3 | 92 | 84 | Stop Look and Listen | 60 | >15 | ■ | | ✂ | | |
| S3 | 93 | 92 | Centering Meditation | 25–40 | U | | ✓ | ✂ | | |
| | | | | | | | | | | |
| S4 | 126 | 73 | Go For the Gold | 30–40 | U | | | | ✎ | |
| S4 | 127 | 82 | Shifting Gears | 15–30 | U | | | | | |
| S4 | 128 | 87 | Open Up | 45–50 | U | ■ | | ✂ | | |
| S4 | 129 | 92 | Biofeedback | 20–30 | U | | | ✂ | | |
| | | | | | | | | | | |
| S5 | 161 | 71 | Affirmation Calendar | 25–30 | U | | | ✂ | ✎ | |
| S5 | 162 | 76 | Eating Under Stress | 40–45 | U | | | ✂ | ✎ | |
| S5 | 163 | 81 | Keep Your Cool | 60–90 | U | ■ | | ✂ | ✎ | |
| S5 | 164 | 91 | Remote Control | 20–30 | U, I | | | | | |
| S5 | 165 | 94 | Yoga | 30–60 | U | | | ✂ | | |

KEY on page 2

© Nancy Loving Tubesing                    Stress and Wellness Reference Guide

| CATEGORY | EXERCISE # | WORKSITE | FAVORITES | INTRODUCTIONS | CHALKTALK | DEMO | RELAXATION | SCRIPT | ACTIVITY | SMALL GROUPS | LARGE GROUP | DISCLOSURE | TRAINER PREP |
|---|---|---|---|---|---|---|---|---|---|---|---|---|---|
| **Stress 1** | | | | | | | | | | | | | |
| | 17 | | | | ● | | ◆ | 99 | | | ✽ | | |
| | 18a | | | | | ➤ | | | | | ✽ | | ❶ |
| | 18b | | | | | ➤ | | | | | ✽ | | |
| | 18c | | | | | | | 99 | | | | | |
| | 19a | | | | | ➤ | | | | | ✽ | | |
| | 19b | | | | | ➤ | | | | | ✽ | | ❷ |
| | 19c | | | | | ➤ | | 99 | | | ✤ | ✽ | | |
| | 20 | | ☆ | | ● | | | | | | ✤ | ✽ | | ❶ |
| **Stress 2** | | | | | | | | | | | | | |
| | 53 | ◆ | ☆ | | ● | | | 99 | | | ✤ | ✽ | ❶ | ❶ |
| | 54 | | | | ● | | | | | | ✤ | ✽ | ❷ | ❷ |
| | 55 | ◆ | | | ● | | | | | | | ✽ | ❶ | ❶ |
| | 56 | | | | ● | | ◆ | | | ◆ | ✤ | ✽ | | |
| | 57 | ◆ | ☆ | | ● | | | 99 | | | | | | ❶ |
| **Stress 3** | | | | | | | | | | | | | |
| | 90 | ◆ | ☆ | | ● | | | | | | ✤ | ✽ | | ❶ |
| | 91 | | | | ● | | ◆ | | | | | ✽ | | |
| | 92 | | | | ● | | | | | | ✤ | ✽ | ❷ | ❷ |
| | 93 | | ☆ | | ● | | ◆ | 99 | | | | ✽ | ❷ | ❶ |
| **Stress 4** | | | | | | | | | | | | | |
| | 126 | ◆ | ☆ | | ● | | | | | | | ✽ | | ❷ |
| | 127 | | | | ● | | | | | ◆ | | ✽ | | ❶ |
| | 128 | | | | ● | | | | | ◆ | ✤ | ✽ | ❷ | ❷ |
| | 129 | | | | ● | ➤ | ◆ | 99 | | | | ✽ | | ❷ |
| **Stress 5** | | | | | | | | | | | | | |
| | 161 | | ☆ | ◆ | ● | | | | | | ✤ | | ❷ | ❶ |
| | 162 | ◆ | | | ● | | | | | | ✤ | ✽ | ❷ | ❷ |
| | 163 | | | | ● | ➤ | | | | ◆ | ✤ | ✽ | ❸ | ❸ |
| | 164 | ◆ | | | ● | ➤ | | | | ◆ | | ✽ | | ❷ |
| | 165 | | | | ● | ➤ | ◆ | | | ◆ | | | | ❷ |

KEY on page 2

©1995 Whole Person Press 210 W Michigan Duluth MN 55802     (800) 247-6789

| VOLUME | EXERCISE # | PAGE # | EXERCISE TITLE | MIN TIME TO MAX TIME | GROUP SIZE | BLACKBOARD | A-V NEEDED | MATERIALS | WORKSHEETS | HANDOUTS |
|---|---|---|---|---|---|---|---|---|---|---|
| | | | **WELLNESS EXPLORATION** | | | | | | | |
| W1 | 6 | 17 | Whole Person Health Appraisal | 20–30 | U, I | | | | ✎ | |
| W1 | 7 | 23 | Four Corners | 15–20 | U | | | ✂ | | |
| W1 | 8 | 25 | Vitality Factors | 30–45 | U, I | ■ | | | ✎ | |
| W1 | 9 | 30 | Wellness Congress | 60–90 | U | ■ | | ✂ | | |
| W1 | 10 | 38 | Health/Illness Images | 90 | U | | | ✂ | | |
| | | | | | | | | | | |
| W2 | 42 | 17 | Investing in Health | 10–15 | U, I | | | | ✎ | |
| W2 | 43 | 22 | My Present Health Status | 30–40 | U | | | | ✎ | |
| W2 | 44 | 26 | Caring Appraisal | 45–60 | U, I | ■ | | | ✎ | |
| W2 | 45 | 35 | Sickness Benefits | 10–15 | U | | | | ✎ | |
| W2 | 46 | 39 | Wheel of Health | 60–90 | 15–150 | ■ | | | ✎ | |
| | | | | | | | | | | |
| W3 | 79 | 17 | Personal Wellness Wheel | 15–20 | U, I | ■ | | | ✎ | |
| W3 | 80 | 22 | Wellness Culture Test | 60–90 | U | ■ | | ✂ | ✎ | |
| W3 | 81 | 29 | Pathology of Normalcy | 5 | U | | | | | |
| W3 | 82 | 32 | Well Cards | 30–45 | U, I | | | | | |
| W3 | 83 | 37 | Health Lifelines | 75–90 | U, I | ■ | | ✂ | ✎ | |
| W3 | 84 | 44 | Stand Up and Be Counted | 15–20 | U | | | | | |
| | | | | | | | | | | |
| W4 | 115 | 17 | Wellness Profile | 15–20 | U | | | | ✎ | |
| W4 | 116 | 23 | Whole Person Potpourri | 60–90 | 40–100 | | | ✂ | | |
| W4 | 117 | 33 | Health and Lifestyle | 60–90 | U | | ✓ | | ✎ | |
| W4 | 118 | 39 | Wellness Philosophy | 20–30 | U | | | | ✎ | |
| W4 | 119 | 44 | Symphony of the Cells | 20–30 | >40 | | | ✂ | | |
| | | | | | | | | | | |
| W5 | 150 | 15 | Family Health Tree | 50–60 | U, I | | | | ✎ | |
| W5 | 151 | 23 | Life Themes | 90 | U, I | | | ✂ | ✎ | |
| W5 | 152 | 33 | Pie Charts | 20–30 | U | ■ | | | ✎ | |
| W5 | 153 | 37 | State Flag | 10–15 | U | | | ✂ | ✎ | |
| W5 | 154 | 40 | Work APGAR | 10–15 | U | | | | ✎ | |

KEY on page 2

| CATEGORY | EXERCISE # | WORKSITE | FAVORITES | INTRODUCTIONS | CHALKTALK | DEMO | RELAXATION | SCRIPT | ACTIVITY | SMALL GROUPS | LARGE GROUP | DISCLOSURE | TRAINER PREP |
|---|---|---|---|---|---|---|---|---|---|---|---|---|---|
| **Wellness 1** | | | | | | | | | | | | | |
| | 6 | ◆ | ☆ | | ● | | | | | ⁘ | ✳ | | |
| | 7 | | | | ● | | | | ◆ | ⁘ | ✳ | ❶ | ❷ |
| | 8 | | | | | | | | | | | | ❶ |
| | 9 | | | | ● | | | | | ⁘ | | | ❷ |
| | 10 | | ☆ | | ● | | | | | ⁘ | ✳ | | |
| **Wellness 2** | | | | | | | | | | | | | |
| | 42 | ◆ | | | ● | | | | | | ✳ | | ❶ |
| | 43 | | | | | | | | ◆ | ⁘ | | ❷ | ❶ |
| | 44 | | ☆ | | ● | | | | | ⁘ | ✳ | ❷ | ❷ |
| | 45 | | | | ● | | | | | | ✳ | | ❶ |
| | 46 | | ☆ | | ● | ➤ | | | | | ✳ | | ❸ |
| **Wellness 3** | | | | | | | | | | | | | |
| | 79 | | ☆ | | ● | | | | | | ✳ | ❶ | ❶ |
| | 80 | ◆ | | | ● | | | | ◆ | ⁘ | ✳ | ❶ | ❷ |
| | 81 | ◆ | | | ● | | | 99 | | | ✳ | | |
| | 82 | | | | ● | | | | ◆ | ⁘ | ✳ | ❶ | ❷ |
| | 83 | | ☆ | | ● | | | | | ⁘ | ✳ | ❷ | ❷ |
| | 84 | | ☆ | | ● | ➤ | | | ◆ | | ✳ | | |
| **Wellness 4** | | | | | | | | | | | | | |
| | 115 | | | | ● | | | | | | | | ❶ |
| | 116 | | ☆ | | | ➤ | | | ◆ | ⁘ | ✳ | | ❷ |
| | 117 | ☆ | | | | ➤ | ◆ | 99 | | ⁘ | | ❷ | ❷ |
| | 118 | | | | ● | | | | ◆ | ⁘ | ✳ | ❶ | ❶ |
| | 119 | | | | ● | ➤ | | | ◆ | ⁘ | ✳ | | ❷ |
| **Wellness 5** | | | | | | | | | | | | | |
| | 150 | | ☆ | | ● | ➤ | | | | ⁘ | | ❷ | ❸ |
| | 151 | | | | ● | | | | | ⁘ | ✳ | ❶ | ❷ |
| | 152 | ◆ | ☆ | | ● | | | | | ⁘ | ✳ | | ❶ |
| | 153 | | | | | | | | | ⁘ | ✳ | | ❶ |
| | 154 | ◆ | | | ● | | | | | ⁘ | ✳ | ❶ | ❶ |

KEY on page 2

©1995  Whole Person Press 210 W Michigan Duluth MN 55802          (800) 247-6789

| VOLUME | EXERCISE # | PAGE # | EXERCISE TITLE | MIN TIME TO MAX TIME | GROUP SIZE | BLACKBOARD | A-V NEEDED | MATERIALS | WORKSHEETS | HANDOUTS |
|---|---|---|---|---|---|---|---|---|---|---|
| | | | **SELF-CARE STRATEGIES** | | | | | | | |
| W1 | 11 | 49 | The Marathon Strategy | 15 | U | ■ | | | ✎ | |
| W1 | 12 | 54 | Daily Rituals | 10–15 | U | | | ✂ | | |
| W1 | 13 | 56 | Letter from the Interior | 20–30 | U, I | | | ✂ | | |
| W1 | 14 | 58 | The Last Meal | 15–30 | U | | | | ✎ | |
| W1 | 15 | 62 | The Exercise Exercise | 15 | U | | ✓ | ✂ | | |
| W1 | 16 | 67 | Sanctuary | 15–30 | U, I | | | | | |
| W1 | 17 | 70 | Marco Polo | 15–20 | U | | ✓ | | ✎ | |
| W1 | 18 | 74 | Discriminating Feeler | 30–45 | U | ■ | | | | |
| W1 | 19 | 81 | Interpersonal Needs | 60–90 | U | ■ | | | ✎ | |
| W1 | 20 | 90 | Irish Sweepstakes | 20–30 | U | | | | ✎ | |
| W1 | 21 | 94 | Spiritual Pilgrimage | 20–30 | U, I | | | ✂ | | |
| | | | | | | | | | | |
| W2 | 47 | 49 | Self-Care Learning Contract | 5–10 | U, I | | | | ✎ | |
| W2 | 48 | 52 | Wish List | 5 | U | | | | ✎ | |
| W2 | 49 | 55 | Annual Physical | 30–45 | U | | | ✂ | | |
| W2 | 50 | 58 | Lunch Duets | 60–120 | U | | | ✂ | | |
| W2 | 51 | 63 | Personal Fitness Check | 60 | 12–30 | ■ | | | ✎ | |
| W2 | 52 | 68 | Medicine Cabinet | 45–60 | 15–40 | | | ✂ | | |
| W2 | 53 | 72 | The Power of Positive Thinking | 5 | U | | | | | |
| W2 | 54 | 75 | Loneliness Locator | 60–90 | 8–12 | ■ | | | ✎ | |
| W2 | 55 | 82 | Compass | 30–60 | U, I | | | ✂ | | |
| W2 | 56 | 85 | Life and Death Questions | 30–60 | U, I | ■ | | ✂ | | |
| W2 | 57 | 89 | Self-Care SOAP | 90 | 12–30 | ■ | | ✂ | ✎ | |
| | | | | | | | | | | |
| W3 | 85 | 49 | Auto/Body Checkup | 15–20 | U | | | | ✎ | |
| W3 | 86 | 55 | Chemical Independence | 25–35 | 12–30 | | | | ✎ | |
| W3 | 87 | 60 | Consciousness-Raising Diet | 10–15 | U, I | ■ | | | | |
| W3 | 88 | 62 | Countdown to Relaxation | 5–10 | U, I | | | | | |
| W3 | 89 | 65 | Fit to be Interviewed | 45 | U, I | | | | ✎ | |

KEY on page 2

| CATEGORY | EXERCISE # | WORKSITE | FAVORITES | INTRODUCTIONS | CHALKTALK | DEMO | RELAXATION | SCRIPT | ACTIVITY | SMALL GROUPS | LARGE GROUP | DISCLOSURE | TRAINER PREP |
|---|---|---|---|---|---|---|---|---|---|---|---|---|---|
| **Wellness 1** | | | | | | | | | | | | | |
| self-care | 11 | ◆ | ☆ | | ● | | | | | | ✳ | | ❷ |
| self-care | 12 | | | | ● | | | | | | ✳ | ❶ | ❶ |
| physical | 13 | | | | | | | | | ✛ | ✳ | ❷ | ❶ |
| eating | 14 | | | | | | | | | ✛ | ✳ | ❷ | ❶ |
| exercise | 15 | ◆ | | | ● | ➤ | | | ◆ | | | | |
| relaxation | 16 | ◆ | | | | ➤ | ◆ | 99 | | | ✳ | | |
| mental | 17 | | ☆ | | | | | | | | ✳ | ❶ | ❷ |
| emotional | 18 | | | | ● | | | | | ✛ | ✳ | ❶ | ❶ |
| interpersonal | 19 | | ☆ | | ● | | | | | ✛ | ✳ | ❶ | ❷ |
| lifestyle | 20 | | | | ● | | | | | ✛ | ✳ | ❶ | ❶ |
| spiritual | 21 | | ☆ | ◆ | ● | | | | | ✛ | | ❷ | ❶ |
| **Wellness 2** | | | | | | | | | | | | | |
| self-care | 47 | ◆ | | | | | | | | ✛ | ✳ | ❷ | ❶ |
| self-care | 48 | | | | | | | | | | | | ❶ |
| physical | 49 | | | | | | | | | ✛ | | ❷ | ❶ |
| eating | 50 | | | | ● | ➤ | | | ◆ | ✛ | ✳ | | ❷ |
| exercise | 51 | ◆ | | | | | | | | | ✳ | | ❶ |
| self-care | 52 | | | | ● | | | | ◆ | ✛ | ✳ | | ❷ |
| mental | 53 | | | | | ➤ | | | ◆ | ✛ | ✳ | | |
| interpersonal | 54 | | | | ● | | | | | | ✳ | ❸ | ❸ |
| lifestyle | 55 | | ☆ | | ● | | | | | ✛ | ✳ | ❷ | ❶ |
| spiritual | 56 | | ☆ | | ● | | | | | ✛ | ✳ | ❷ | ❷ |
| self-care | 57 | ◆ | | | ● | ➤ | | | ◆ | ✛ | ✳ | ❶ | ❸ |
| **Wellness 3** | | | | | | | | | | | | | |
| self-care | 85 | | | | ● | | | | | ✛ | ✳ | ❶ | ❶ |
| self-care | 86 | | | | | | | | | ✛ | ✳ | ❶ | ❶ |
| eating | 87 | | ☆ | | ● | | | | | | | | |
| relaxation | 88 | | ☆ | | ● | | ◆ | 99 | | | ✳ | | |
| exercise | 89 | | | | | | | | | | ✳ | | ❷ |

KEY on page 2

©1995 Whole Person Press 210 W Michigan Duluth MN 55802 (800) 247-6789

| VOLUME | EXERCISE # | PAGE # | EXERCISE TITLE | MIN TIME TO MAX TIME | GROUP SIZE | BLACKBOARD | A-V NEEDED | MATERIALS | WORKSHEETS | |
|--------|-----------|--------|----------------|---------------------|------------|------------|-----------|-----------|------------|---|
| | | | **SELF-CARE STRATEGIES** | | | | | | | |
| W3 | 90 | 70 | Journal to Music | 60–90 | U | | ✓ | ✀ | | |
| W3 | 91 | 76 | Openness and Intimacy | 50–60 | 10–40 | ■ | | | ✐ | |
| W3 | 92 | 82 | That's the Spirit! | 10–15 | U | | | | ✐ | |
| W3 | 93 | 86 | Footloose and Fancy Free | 10–20 | U | | | | | |
| W3 | 94 | 90 | Polaroid Perspectives | 30–50 | U, I | | | ✀ | ✐ | |
| | | | | | | | | | | |
| W4 | 120 | 49 | Decades | 15–20 | U | | | | ✐ | |
| W4 | 121 | 52 | Take a Walk! | 45–60 | U | ■ | | ✀ | | |
| W4 | 122 | 59 | Calorie Counter's Prayer | 10–15 | U | | | | ✐ | |
| W4 | 123 | 62 | Self-Esteem Grid | 45–50 | U | | | | ✐ | |
| W4 | 124 | 68 | Wellness Meditation | 15 | U | | ✓ | | | |
| W4 | 125 | 71 | Expanding Your Circles | 20–30 | U | | | | | |
| W4 | 126 | 75 | Depth Finder | 30–45 | U | | | ✀ | ✐ | |
| W4 | 127 | 79 | Let's Play | 40–45 | 20–40 | ■ | | | | |
| W4 | 128 | 85 | Job Motivators | 40–50 | U | ■ | | | ✐ | |
| W4 | 129 | 93 | Information is Not Enough | 20–30 | U | | | ✀ | | |
| | | | | | | | | | | |
| W5 | 155 | 45 | Values and Self-Care Choices | 20–30 | U | | | | ✐ | |
| W5 | 156 | 49 | Assertive Consumer | 40–50 | U | | | ✀ | ✐ | |
| W5 | 157 | 56 | Mealtime Meditation | 10–15 | U, I | | ✓ | | | |
| W5 | 158 | 61 | Healthy Exercise | 20–60 | U | | ✓ | | ✐ | |
| W5 | 159 | 63 | Imagery for a Healthy Heart | 10–15 | U | | ✓ | | | |
| W5 | 160 | 68 | Seventh Inning Stretch | 5–10 | U | | | | | |
| W5 | 161 | 71 | Mental Health Index | 30–45 | U | | | ✀ | ✐ | |
| W5 | 162 | 76 | Seven Ways of Knowing | 60–90 | U | | | ✀ | ✐ | |
| W5 | 163 | 85 | Relationship Report Card | 30–40 | U, I | | | ✀ | ✐ | |
| W5 | 164 | 89 | Spiritual Fingerprint | 60 | U | ■ | | ✀ | | |
| W5 | 165 | 93 | Leisure Pursuits | 20–30 | U | ■ | | | ✐ | |
| | | | | | | | | | | |

KEY on page 2

| CATEGORY | EXERCISE # | WORKSITE | FAVORITES | INTRODUCTIONS | CHALKTALK | DEMO | RELAXATION | SCRIPT | ACTIVITY | SMALL GROUPS | LARGE GROUP | DISCLOSURE | TRAINER PREP |
|---|---|---|---|---|---|---|---|---|---|---|---|---|---|
| **Wellness 3** | | | | | | | | | | | | | |
| emotional | 90 | | ☆ | | ● | | ◆ | | | | ✳ | ❷ | ❷ |
| interpersonal | 91 | | ☆ | | ● | | | | | ✛ | ✳ | ❷ | ❷ |
| spiritual | 92 | ◆ | | | ● | | | | | | ✳ | | ❶ |
| lifestyle | 93 | | ☆ | | ● | | | 99 | | ✛ | | ❷ | |
| self-care | 94 | | ☆ | | ● | | | | | ✛ | ✳ | ❷ | ❷ |
| **Wellness 4** | | | | | | | | | | | | | |
| self-care | 120 | | | | | | | | | ✛ | | ❶ | ❶ |
| exercise | 121 | ◆ | ☆ | | ● | ➤ | ◆ | | ◆ | ✛ | ✳ | ❶ | ❷ |
| eating | 122 | | | | | | | 99 | | | ✳ | ❶ | ❶ |
| emotional | 123 | | ☆ | | ● | | | | | ✛ | ✳ | ❶ | ❷ |
| relaxation | 124 | | | | ● | | ◆ | 99 | | | ✳ | | ❶ |
| interpersonal | 125 | | | | ● | | | | | ✛ | ✳ | ❷ | ❷ |
| spiritual | 126 | | | | ● | | | | | ✛ | ✳ | ❶ | ❷ |
| lifestyle | 127 | | ☆ | | ● | ➤ | | 99 | ◆ | ✛ | ✳ | ❶ | ❷ |
| mental | 128 | ◆ | | | ● | | | | | ✛ | ✳ | ❷ | ❷ |
| self-care | 129 | | ☆ | | ● | | | | | | ✳ | | ❶ |
| **Wellness 5** | | | | | | | | | | | | | |
| self-care | 155 | | | | ● | | | | | ✛ | ✳ | ❶ | ❶ |
| self-care | 156 | | | ◆ | ● | | | | | ✛ | | ❷ | |
| eating | 157 | | ☆ | | ● | | ◆ | 99 | | | ✳ | | ❶ |
| exercise | 158 | ◆ | | | | | ◆ | | | ✛ | | | ❶ |
| physical | 159 | | | | ● | | ◆ | 99 | | | | | ❶ |
| relaxation | 160 | | | | | | | | ◆ | | ✳ | | |
| emotional | 161 | | | | ● | | | | | | ✳ | | ❷ |
| mental | 162 | ◆ | | | ● | ➤ | | | | ✛ | ✳ | | ❸ |
| interpersonal | 163 | | | | ● | | | | | ✛ | | | ❶ |
| spiritual | 164 | | ☆ | | ● | | | | | ✛ | | ❶ | ❷ |
| lifestyle | 165 | ◆ | | | | | | | | ✛ | ✳ | | ❶ |

KEY on page 2

©1995  Whole Person Press 210 W Michigan Duluth MN 55802     (800) 247-6789

| VOLUME | EXERCISE # | PAGE # | EXERCISE TITLE | MIN TIME TO MAX TIME | GROUP SIZE | BLACKBOARD | A-V NEEDED | MATERIALS | WORKSHEETS | HANDOUTS |
|---|---|---|---|---|---|---|---|---|---|---|
| | | | **PLANNING & CLOSURE** | | | | | | | |
| S1 | 21 | 89 | Getting Out of My Box | 60–90 | U, I | | | | ✎ | |
| S1 | 22 | 102 | One Step at a Time | 20–30 | U, I | | | | ✎ | |
| S1 | 23 | 108 | Postscript | 15 | U, I | | | ✂ | | |
| S1 | 24 | 110 | Coping Skill Affirmation | 60 | U | | | ✂ | | |
| | | | | | | | | | | |
| S2 | 58 | 97 | Personal/Professional Review | 10–15 | U | | | | | |
| S2 | 59 | 98 | Manager of the Year | 45–60 | 12–25 | | | ✂ | ✎ | ⌐ |
| S2 | 60 | 102 | Goals, Obstacles and Actions | 30–60 | U, I | | | ✂ | ✎ | |
| S2 | 61 | 108 | 25 Words or Less | 10–15 | 8–40 | | | ✂ | | |
| S2 | 62 | 110 | Stress and Coping Journal | 5–10 | U, I | | | | | ⌐ |
| | | | | | | | | | | |
| S3 | 94 | 97 | Closing Formation | 10–30 | >16 | | | | | |
| S3 | 95 | 100 | Exit Interview | 20–30 | U | | | | | ⌐ |
| S3 | 96 | 104 | Recipe for Success with Stress | 25–30 | U | | | | ✎ | |
| S3 | 97 | 107 | My Stress Reduction Program | 20–30 | U | | | | ✎ | |
| S3 | 98 | 110 | Change Pentagon | 15–30 | U, I | | | | ✎ | |
| | | | | | | | | | | |
| S4 | 130 | 97 | ABCDEFG Planner | 20–30 | U | | | | ✎ | |
| S4 | 131 | 102 | So What? | 10–15 | U, I | | | | ✎ | |
| S4 | 132 | 105 | Group Banner | 15–25 | U | | | ✂ | | |
| S4 | 133 | 107 | Pat on the Back | 20–30 | 6–8 | | | ✂ | | |
| S4 | 134 | 112 | Dear Me P.S. | 10–15 | U | | | ✂ | | |
| | | | | | | | | | | |
| S5 | 166 | 99 | Five and Ten | 10–15 | U, I | | | ✂ | | |
| S5 | 167 | 101 | Go Fly a Kite | 10–20 | U | | | | ✎ | |
| S5 | 168 | 105 | Hope Chest | 15–20 | U | | | | ✎ | |
| S5 | 169 | 108 | Key Learning | 5–10 | U | ■ | | | ✎ | |
| S5 | 170 | 111 | Stress Examiner | 20–30 | U | | | ✂ | | |
| | | | | | | | | | | |

KEY on page 2

| CATEGORY | EXERCISE # | WORKSITE | FAVORITES | INTRODUCTIONS | CHALKTALK | DEMO | RELAXATION | SCRIPT | ACTIVITY | SMALL GROUPS | LARGE GROUP | DISCLOSURE | TRAINER PREP |
|---|---|---|---|---|---|---|---|---|---|---|---|---|---|
| **Stress 1** | | | | | | | | | | | | | |
| | 21 | | ☆ | | ● | | | 99 | | ✣ | ✱ | ❷ | ❷ |
| | 22 | | | | | | | | | | ✱ | | ❶ |
| | 23 | | | | | | | | | | | | ❶ |
| | 24 | | | | | | | | | | | ❶ | ❷ |
| **Stress 2** | | | | | | | | | | | | | |
| | 58 | | | | | | | | | | ✱ | ❶ | |
| | 59 | ◆ | | | | | | | ◆ | ✣ | | ❷ | ❷ |
| | 60 | | ☆ | | | | | | | | | | ❶ |
| | 61 | | | | | | | | | | ✱ | ❶ | ❶ |
| | 62 | | | | | | | | | | | | ❶ |
| **Stress 3** | | | | | | | | | | | | | |
| | 94 | ◆ | ☆ | | | | | | | ✣ | | ❶ | ❶ |
| | 95 | | | | | | | | | ✣ | ✱ | ❷ | ❶ |
| | 96 | | | | | | | | | | ✱ | ❶ | ❶ |
| | 97 | ◆ | | | | | | | | | ✱ | ❶ | ❶ |
| | 98 | | ☆ | | | | | | | ✣ | ✱ | ❶ | ❶ |
| **Stress 4** | | | | | | | | | | | | | |
| | 130 | | | | | | | | | | ✱ | | ❶ |
| | 131 | | ☆ | | | | | | | | ✱ | ❶ | ❶ |
| | 132 | | | | | | | | ◆ | ✣ | ✱ | | ❷ |
| | 133 | ◆ | | | | | | | ◆ | ✣ | ✱ | ❷ | ❷ |
| | 134 | | ☆ | | | | | | | | ✱ | ❶ | |
| **Stress 5** | | | | | | | | | | | | | |
| | 166 | | ☆ | | | | | | | ✣ | ✱ | ❷ | |
| | 167 | | | | ● | | | | | ✣ | | ❷ | ❶ |
| | 168 | | | | | | | | | ✣ | | ❶ | ❶ |
| | 169 | ◆ | | | | | | | | ✣ | | ❶ | ❶ |
| | 170 | | | | | | | | | | ✱ | ❶ | ❶ |

KEY on page 2

©1995  Whole Person Press 210 W Michigan Duluth MN 55802       (800) 247-6789

| VOLUME | EXERCISE # | PAGE # | EXERCISE TITLE | MIN TIME TO MAX TIME | GROUP SIZE | BLACKBOARD | A-V NEEDED | MATERIALS | WORKSHEETS | HANDOUTS |
|---|---|---|---|---|---|---|---|---|---|---|
| | | | **PLANNING & CLOSURE** | | | | | | | |
| W1 | 22 | 97 | Shoulds, Wants, Wills | 15–20 | U, I | | | ✂ | | |
| W1 | 23 | 100 | What Do You Need? | 10–15 | U, I | | | | ✐ | |
| W1 | 24 | 104 | Real to Ideal | 10–15 | U, I | | | | ✐ | |
| W1 | 25 | 110 | Personal Prescription | 5–10 | U, I | | | | ✐ | |
| W1 | 26 | 112 | Meet the New Me | 10–15 | 10–15 | | | ✂ | | |
| | | | | | | | | | | |
| W2 | 58 | 97 | What Next? | 10–15 | U | | | | | |
| W2 | 59 | 98 | Roundup Revisited | 1–2 | <25 | | | | | |
| W2 | 60 | 99 | Cleaning Up My Act | 30–45 | U, I | ■ | | ✂ | ✐ | |
| W2 | 61 | 106 | One-a-Day Plan | 20–30 | U, I | ■ | | | ✐ | |
| W2 | 62 | 109 | Vital Signs | 10–15 | U | | | ✂ | ✐ | |
| | | | | | | | | | | |
| W3 | 95 | 97 | Closing Statements | 10–30 | U | | | | ✐ | |
| W3 | 96 | 100 | Daily Wellness Graph | 20–30 | 6–12 | | | | ✐ | |
| W3 | 97 | 106 | Fortune Cookies | 15–20 | U | ■ | | ✂ | | |
| W3 | 98 | 109 | Health Report Card | 25–30 | U | | | ✂ | | |
| | | | | | | | | | | |
| W4 | 130 | 97 | Beat the Odds | 10–15 | U | | | ✂ | ✐ | |
| W4 | 131 | 100 | Discoveries | 20–30 | U | | | ✂ | ✐ | |
| W4 | 132 | 106 | Gifts | 5–15 | U | | | ✂ | | |
| W4 | 133 | 108 | Work of Art | 30 | U | | | ✂ | | |
| W4 | 134 | 111 | Whisper Circle | 10–15 | U | | | | | |
| | | | | | | | | | | |
| W5 | 166 | 97 | Commercial Success | 15–20 | 15–30 | | | | | |
| W5 | 167 | 99 | If . . . Then | 15–20 | U | ■ | | | ✐ | |
| W5 | 168 | 102 | Just for Today | 15–20 | U | | | | ✐ | |
| W5 | 169 | 106 | Self-Care Bouquet | 20–30 | U | | | ✂ | | |
| W5 | 170 | 110 | Take the Pledge | 10–15 | U | | | | ✐ | |

KEY on page 2

| CATEGORY | EXERCISE # | WORKSITE | FAVORITES | INTRODUCTIONS | CHALKTALK | DEMO | RELAXATION | SCRIPT | ACTIVITY | SMALL GROUPS | LARGE GROUP | DISCLOSURE | TRAINER PREP |
|---|---|---|---|---|---|---|---|---|---|---|---|---|---|
| **Wellness 1** | | | | | | | | | | | | | |
| | 22 | ◆ | | | ● | | | | | ✣ | | ❶ | ❶ |
| | 23 | | | | | | | | | | ✳ | | ❶ |
| | 24 | | | | | | | | | | ✳ | ❶ | ❶ |
| | 25 | ◆ | ☆ | | | | | | | | | | ❶ |
| | 26 | | ☆ | ◆ | | | | | | ✣ | | ❷ | |
| **Wellness 2** | | | | | | | | | | | | | |
| | 58 | | | | | | ◆ | | | | | | |
| | 59 | ◆ | | | ● | | | | | | ✳ | ❶ | |
| | 60 | | ☆ | | ● | | | | | | | | ❸ |
| | 61 | | ☆ | | ● | | | | | | ✳ | | ❶ |
| | 62 | ◆ | | | | | | | | ✣ | ✳ | ❷ | ❶ |
| **Wellness 3** | | | | | | | | | | | | | |
| | 95 | ◆ | | | | | | | | | ✳ | ❶ | ❶ |
| | 96 | ◆ | | | ● | | | | | | ✳ | | ❶ |
| | 97 | | | | | | | | ◆ | ✣ | ✳ | ❶ | ❷ |
| | 98 | | | | | | | | | ✣ | ✳ | ❷ | ❶ |
| **Wellness 4** | | | | | | | | | | | | | |
| | 130 | | ☆ | | ● | | | | | | ✳ | ❶ | ❶ |
| | 131 | ◆ | | | ● | | | | | | ✳ | ❶ | ❷ |
| | 132 | | | | | | | | | ✣ | ✳ | ❷ | ❷ |
| | 133 | | | | | | | | ◆ | ✣ | | ❶ | ❸ |
| | 134 | | ☆ | | | | | | | ✣ | ✳ | ❷ | |
| **Wellness 5** | | | | | | | | | | | | | |
| | 166 | | ☆ | | | | | | | ✣ | ✳ | | |
| | 167 | ◆ | | | | | | | | ✣ | | ❶ | ❶ |
| | 168 | | | | | | 99 | | | | | ❶ | ❶ |
| | 169 | | | | ● | | | | | ✣ | | ❶ | ❶ |
| | 170 | | | | | | | | | ✣ | | | ❶ |

KEY on page 2

©1995  Whole Person Press 210 W Michigan Duluth MN 55802     (800) 247-6789

| VOLUME | EXERCISE # | PAGE # | EXERCISE TITLE | MIN TIME TO MAX TIME | GROUP SIZE | BLACKBOARD | A-V NEEDED | MATERIALS | WORKSHEETS | HANDOUTS |
|---|---|---|---|---|---|---|---|---|---|---|
| | | | **GROUP ENERGIZERS** | | | | | | | |
| S1 | 25 | 113 | Boo-Down | 5 | >50 | | | ✂ | | |
| S1 | 26 | 116 | Breath-less | 2 | U | | | | | |
| S1 | 27 | 117 | Catastrophe Game | 10–15 | U | | | | | |
| S1 | 28 | 119 | Fruit Basket Upset | 2–5 | U | | | | | |
| S1 | 29 | 120 | Get Off My Back! | 2 | U | | | | | |
| S1 | 30 | 121 | Hot Potato Problem | 15–20 | U | | ✓ | ✂ | | |
| S1 | 31 | 124 | Pulling Strings | 5–10 | U | | | | | |
| S1 | 32 | 125 | Singalong 2 | 2–5 | U | ■ | | | | ▢ |
| S1 | 33 | 127 | Stress Spending | 10–30 | U, I | | | ✂ | | |
| S1 | 34 | 129 | S-T-R-E-T-C-H | 5 | U | | | ✂ | | |
| S1 | 35 | 131 | Ten Great Trips on Foot | 5 | U | | | | | |
| S1 | 36 | 133 | Tension Hurts | 5 | U | | | | | |
| | | | | | | | | | | |
| S2 | 63 | 113 | The Garden | 5 | U | | | | | |
| S2 | 64 | 115 | Hand-to-Hand Contact | 10 | U | | | | | ▢ |
| S2 | 65 | 118 | Helpers Anonymous | 5 | >20 | | | ✂ | | ▢ |
| S2 | 66 | 120 | Musical Movement | 10–15 | U | | ✓ | ✂ | | |
| S2 | 67 | 122 | Round of Applause | 2 | U | | | | | |
| S2 | 68 | 123 | Seaweed and Oak | 5–10 | U | | | | | |
| S2 | 69 | 125 | Stress Stretchers | 5–10 | U | | | ✂ | | |
| S2 | 70 | 127 | Target Practice | 10 | U | | | | | |
| S2 | 71 | 129 | Ten-Second Break | 5 | U | | | | | ▢ |
| S2 | 72 | 131 | Treasure Chest | 15–20 | U | | | | | |
| | | | | | | | | | | |
| S3 | 99 | 113 | Kicking Your Stress Can-Can | 5 | U | | ✓ | | | |
| S3 | 100 | 114 | Chinese Swing | 10 | U | | | ✂ | | |
| S3 | 101 | 116 | Clouds to Sunshine | 3–5 | U | | | ✂ | | |
| S3 | 102 | 118 | Create a Singalong | 10–15 | U | ■ | | | | |
| S3 | 103 | 120 | Groans and Moans | 5–15 | U | | ✓ | ✂ | | |

KEY on page 2

| CATEGORY | EXERCISE # | WORKSITE | FAVORITES | INTRODUCTIONS | CHALKTALK | DEMO | RELAXATION | SCRIPT | ACTIVITY | SMALL GROUPS | LARGE GROUP | DISCLOSURE | TRAINER PREP |
|---|---|---|---|---|---|---|---|---|---|---|---|---|---|
| **Stress 1** | | | | | | | | | | | | | |
| | 25 | | ☆ | | | ➤ | | | ◆ | | ✳ | | ❶ |
| | 26 | | | | ● | ➤ | | | | | ✳ | | |
| | 27 | | | | ● | | | | | ✜ | | | |
| | 28 | | ☆ | | | | | | ◆ | | ✳ | | |
| | 29 | | | | | | | | | | ✳ | | |
| | 30 | | | | | ➤ | | | ◆ | | | | ❶ |
| | 31 | ◆ | | | | | ◆ | | ◆ | | ✳ | | |
| | 32 | | | | | | | | | | ✳ | | ❶ |
| | 33 | | | | | | | | ◆ | | ✳ | | ❶ |
| | 34 | | | | ● | | | 99 | ◆ | | ✳ | | |
| | 35 | | ☆ | | | | | 99 | ◆ | | ✳ | | |
| | 36 | | | | ● | ➤ | | | ◆ | | ✳ | | |
| **Stress 2** | | | | | | | | | | | | | |
| | 63 | | ☆ | | ● | | | 99 | | | | | |
| | 64 | | | | | | ◆ | | ◆ | ✜ | ✳ | | ❶ |
| | 65 | | | ◆ | | | | | ◆ | | | | ❶ |
| | 66 | | | | | | ◆ | | ◆ | | | | ❶ |
| | 67 | ◆ | | | | ➤ | | | ◆ | | ✳ | | |
| | 68 | | | | | ➤ | | 99 | ◆ | | ✳ | | |
| | 69 | | | | | ➤ | | | ◆ | | ✳ | | ❶ |
| | 70 | | | | | ➤ | | | ◆ | | ✳ | | |
| | 71 | | | | | | ◆ | | ◆ | | ✳ | | ❶ |
| | 72 | | | | | | ◆ | 99 | | ✜ | | ❶ | |
| **Stress 3** | | | | | | | | | | | | | |
| | 99 | | | | | | | | ◆ | | ✳ | | ❶ |
| | 100 | | | | | | ◆ | 99 | ◆ | | ✳ | | |
| | 101 | | | | | | ◆ | 99 | ◆ | | ✳ | | ❶ |
| | 102 | | | | | | | | | ✜ | ✳ | | |
| | 103 | | ☆ | | ● | | ◆ | | | | ✳ | | |

KEY on page 2

©1995  Whole Person Press 210 W Michigan Duluth MN 55802     (800) 247-6789

| VOLUME | EXERCISE # | PAGE # | EXERCISE TITLE | MIN TIME TO MAX TIME | GROUP SIZE | BLACKBOARD | A-V NEEDED | MATERIALS | WORKSHEETS | HANDOUTS |
|---|---|---|---|---|---|---|---|---|---|---|
| | | | **GROUP ENERGIZERS** | | | | | | | |
| S3 | 104 | 122 | Tug of War | 5–10 | >8 | | | ✂ | | |
| S3 | 105 | 124 | Warm Hands | 5–10 | U | | | | | |
| S3 | 106 | 126 | What's the Hurry? | 5 | U | | | | | |
| S3 | 107 | 129 | You're Not Listening | 5–10 | U | | | | | |
| S3 | 108 | 131 | Pushing My Buttons | 10–15 | U | | | | | |
| | | | | | | | | | | |
| S4 | 135 | 113 | Giraffe | 5 | U | | | | | |
| S4 | 136 | 115 | Hot Tub | 8 | U | | ✓ | | | |
| S4 | 137 | 118 | How to Swim with Sharks | 5 | U | | | | | |
| S4 | 138 | 120 | Human Knots | 5–10 | U | | | | | |
| S4 | 139 | 122 | Merry-Go-Round | 5–15 | 8–20 | | | ✂ | | |
| S4 | 140 | 124 | Microwave | 2 | U | | | | | |
| S4 | 141 | 126 | The Mustard Seed | 5 | U | | | | | |
| S4 | 142 | 128 | Revitalize Your Eyes | 2–5 | U | | | | | |
| S4 | 143 | 130 | Sigh of Relief | 3–5 | U | | | | | |
| S4 | 144 | 132 | Snap, Crackle, Pop | 5–10 | U | | | | | |
| | | | | | | | | | | |
| S5 | 171 | 113 | Anti-Stress Coffee Break | 10–15 | U | ■ | | ✂ | | |
| S5 | 172 | 115 | Breath Prayer | 8–10 | U | | | | | |
| S5 | 173 | 118 | Cobra | 5 | U | | | ✂ | | |
| S5 | 174 | 120 | Hand Dancing | 10 | >8 | | ✓ | | | |
| S5 | 175 | 122 | Humming Breath | 3–5 | U | | | | | |
| S5 | 176 | 124 | Stress Squeezers | 10–15 | U | | | ✂ | | |
| S5 | 177 | 126 | Superman | 5–10 | U | | | ✂ | | ⌐ |
| S5 | 178 | 129 | Too Bad! | 10–15 | U | | | | | |
| S5 | 179 | 131 | Trouble Bubbles | 5–10 | U, I | | ✓ | | | |
| S5 | 180 | 133 | Try, Try Again | 5 | U | | | | | |
| | | | | | | | | | | |
| | | | | | | | | | | |

KEY on page 2

© Nancy Loving Tubesing

| CATEGORY | EXERCISE # | WORKSITE | FAVORITES | INTRODUCTIONS | CHALKTALK | DEMO | RELAXATION | SCRIPT | ACTIVITY | SMALL GROUPS | LARGE GROUP | DISCLOSURE | TRAINER PREP |
|---|---|---|---|---|---|---|---|---|---|---|---|---|---|
| **Stress 3** | | | | | | | | | | | | | |
| | 104 | | | | | ➤ | | | ◆ | ✣ | ✳ | | |
| | 105 | | | | | | ◆ | 99 | | | | | |
| | 106 | | ☆ | | | | | 99 | | | ✳ | | |
| | 107 | ◆ | | | | ➤ | | | ◆ | ✣ | | | |
| | 108 | | | | | | ◆ | 99 | ◆ | | ✳ | | ❶ |
| **Stress 4** | | | | | | | | | | | | | |
| | 135 | | | | | | ◆ | 99 | ◆ | | | | |
| | 136 | | | | | | ◆ | 99 | | | | | ❶ |
| | 137 | ◆ | | | | | | 99 | | | | | |
| | 138 | | | | ● | ➤ | | | ◆ | ✣ | | | |
| | 139 | | | | | ➤ | | | ◆ | | ✳ | | ❶ |
| | 140 | | | | | | | | ◆ | | | | |
| | 141 | | | | | | | 99 | | | ✳ | | |
| | 142 | | | | ● | | ◆ | | ◆ | | | | |
| | 143 | | | | ● | | ◆ | | ◆ | | | | |
| | 144 | | ☆ | | ● | | ◆ | | ◆ | ✣ | ✳ | | |
| **Stress 5** | | | | | | | | | | | | | |
| | 171 | ◆ | | | | | | 99 | ◆ | | | | ❷ |
| | 172 | | | | ● | | ◆ | 99 | | | ✳ | | |
| | 173 | | | | | ➤ | ◆ | 99 | ◆ | | | | |
| | 174 | | | | | | | | ◆ | ✣ | ✳ | ❷ | |
| | 175 | | ☆ | | ● | ➤ | ◆ | | ◆ | | ✳ | | |
| | 176 | ◆ | | | ● | | | | ◆ | ✣ | ✳ | ❶ | ❸ |
| | 177 | ◆ | | | ● | | | | | ✣ | | ❶ | ❶ |
| | 178 | | | | ● | | | | ◆ | ✣ | ✳ | ❶ | |
| | 179 | | | | | | ◆ | 99 | | | | | |
| | 180 | ◆ | ☆ | | ● | | | 99 | | | | | |

KEY on page 2

©1995  Whole Person Press 210 W Michigan Duluth MN 55802          (800) 247-6789

| VOLUME | EXERCISE # | PAGE # | EXERCISE TITLE | MIN TIME TO MAX TIME | GROUP SIZE | BLACKBOARD | A-V NEEDED | MATERIALS | WORKSHEETS | HANDOUTS |
|---|---|---|---|---|---|---|---|---|---|---|
| | | | **GROUP ENERGIZERS** | | | | | | | |
| W1 | 27 | 115 | 60-Second Tension Tamers | 1 | U | | | | | |
| W1 | 28 | 117 | The Big Myth | 2 | U | | | | | |
| W1 | 29 | 119 | Breathing Meditation | 1–2 | U | | | | | ☐ |
| W1 | 30 | 121 | Grabwell Grommet | 5 | U | | | | | |
| W1 | 31 | 123 | Group Backrub | 2–5 | U | | | | | |
| W1 | 32 | 125 | Megaphone | 5–10 | U | | | | | ☐ |
| W1 | 33 | 127 | Noontime Energizers | 5–10 | U | | | ✎ | | |
| W1 | 34 | 131 | Red Rover | 5–15 | U | | | ✂ | | |
| W1 | 35 | 132 | Singalong | 2–5 | U | ■ | | | | |
| W1 | 36 | 133 | Slogans & Bumper Stickers | 10–15 | U | | | ✂ | | |
| | | | | | | | | | | |
| W2 | 63 | 113 | Body Scanning | 2–3 | U | | | | | |
| W2 | 64 | 115 | Cheers! | 10–15 | U | | | | | |
| W2 | 65 | 116 | Exercises for the Sedentary | 3–5 | U | | | | | |
| W2 | 66 | 118 | Fingertip Face Massage | 10–15 | U | | ✓ | | | |
| W2 | 67 | 121 | Good Morning World | 3–5 | U | | ✓ | | | |
| W2 | 68 | 123 | I'm Depressed! | 2–5 | U | | | | | |
| W2 | 69 | 125 | Take a Deep Breath | 10 | U | | | | | |
| W2 | 70 | 128 | Up, Up and Away | 2–5 | U | | | | | |
| W2 | 71 | 130 | Working Coffee Break | 10–15 | U | | | | | |
| W2 | 72 | 132 | You Asked for It | 4–10 | U | | | | | |
| | | | | | | | | | | |
| W3 | 99 | 113 | 50 Excuses for a Closed Mind | 5–15 | U | | | | | ☐ |
| W3 | 100 | 116 | Breathing Elements | 5 | U | | | | | |
| W3 | 101 | 118 | The Feelings Factory | 2–3 | U | | | | | |
| W3 | 102 | 120 | Limericks | 15–20 | U | | | ✎ | | |
| W3 | 103 | 123 | Balancing Act | 5–10 | U | | | | | |
| W3 | 104 | 124 | Outrageous Episodes | 5–10 | >30 | | | ✂ | | |
| W3 | 105 | 126 | Say the Magic Word | 5–10 | U | | | ✂ | | |

KEY on page 2

| CATEGORY | EXERCISE # | WORKSITE | FAVORITES | INTRODUCTIONS | CHALKTALK | DEMO | RELAXATION | SCRIPT | ACTIVITY | SMALL GROUPS | LARGE GROUP | DISCLOSURE | TRAINER PREP |
|---|---|---|---|---|---|---|---|---|---|---|---|---|---|
| **Wellness 1** | | | | | | | | | | | | | |
| | 27 | ◆ | | | | ➤ | ◆ | | ◆ | | | | |
| | 28 | ◆ | | | | ➤ | | | ◆ | | ✻ | | |
| | 29 | | | | | | ◆ | 99 | | | | | ❶ |
| | 30 | | | | | | | 99 | | | | | |
| | 31 | | | | | | ◆ | | ◆ | | ✻ | | |
| | 32 | | | | | | | | ◆ | | ✻ | | |
| | 33 | ◆ | | | ● | | | | | | ✻ | | ❶ |
| | 34 | | | | | | | | ◆ | | | | |
| | 35 | | ☆ | | | | | | | | | | ❶ |
| | 36 | ◆ | ☆ | | | | | | ◆ | ✛ | ✻ | | ❶ |
| **Wellness 2** | | | | | | | | | | | | | |
| | 63 | ◆ | | | | | ◆ | 99 | | | ✻ | | |
| | 64 | ◆ | | | | | | | ◆ | ✛ | ✻ | | |
| | 65 | ◆ | | | ● | | ◆ | | ◆ | | | | |
| | 66 | ◆ | | | | | ◆ | 99 | ◆ | | ✻ | | ❶ |
| | 67 | | ☆ | | | | ◆ | 99 | ◆ | | | | ❶ |
| | 68 | | ☆ | | | ➤ | | | ◆ | | ✻ | | |
| | 69 | ◆ | | | ● | | ◆ | 99 | | | | | |
| | 70 | ◆ | | | | | ◆ | | ◆ | | ✻ | | |
| | 71 | ◆ | | | | | | | ◆ | ✛ | ✻ | | ❷ |
| | 72 | | | | | ➤ | | | ◆ | ✛ | ✻ | ❷ | |
| **Wellness 3** | | | | | | | | | | | | | |
| | 99 | ◆ | | ● | | ➤ | | | ◆ | | ✻ | | |
| | 100 | | | | | | ◆ | 99 | ◆ | | | | |
| | 101 | | | | | ➤ | | 99 | ◆ | | ✻ | ❶ | |
| | 102 | | ☆ | | | | | | | ✛ | ✻ | | ❶ |
| | 103 | ◆ | | | | ➤ | | | ◆ | ✛ | ✻ | | |
| | 104 | | | | | | | | ◆ | | ✻ | | ❶ |
| | 105 | | | | | | | | | | ✻ | | ❶ |

KEY on page 2

©1995  Whole Person Press 210 W Michigan Duluth MN 55802          (800) 247-6789

| VOLUME | EXERCISE # | PAGE # | EXERCISE TITLE | MIN TIME TO MAX TIME | GROUP SIZE | BLACKBOARD | A-V NEEDED | MATERIALS | WORKSHEETS | HANDOUTS |
|--------|-----------|--------|----------------|----------------------|-----------|------------|-----------|-----------|-----------|----------|
| | | | **GROUP ENERGIZERS** | | | | | | | |
| W3 | 106 | 128 | Standing Ovation | 3 | >25 | | | | | |
| W3 | 107 | 130 | Waves | 5–10 | U | | | | | |
| W3 | 108 | 132 | Weather Report | 5–10 | U | | | | | |
| | | | | | | | | | | |
| W4 | 135 | 113 | 12 Days of Wellness | 5 | U | ■ | | | | |
| W4 | 136 | 115 | All Ears | 5 | U | | | | | |
| W4 | 137 | 116 | As the Seasons Turn | 5 | U | | | | | |
| W4 | 138 | 118 | Clapdance | 5–10 | >25 | | | | | |
| W4 | 139 | 121 | Fit as a Fiddle | 5 | U | | | | | |
| W4 | 140 | 123 | Joke Around | 5 | U | | | | | |
| W4 | 141 | 125 | New Sick Leave Policy | 5 | U | | | | | |
| W4 | 142 | 127 | On Purpose | 10 | U | | ✂ | | | |
| W4 | 143 | 129 | Sensory Relaxation | 5–10 | U | | ✓ | | | |
| W4 | 144 | 132 | Twenty Reasons | 5 | U | | | | | |
| | | | | | | | | | | |
| W5 | 171 | 113 | Choose Wellness Anyway | 3–5 | U | | | | | ▢ |
| W5 | 172 | 115 | Cleansing Breath | 3–5 | U | | | | | |
| W5 | 173 | 117 | For the Health of It | 5–10 | U | | ✓ | | | |
| W5 | 174 | 119 | Healthy Singalong | 3–5 | U | | | | | ▢ |
| W5 | 175 | 121 | Ludicrous Workshops | 15–20 | U | | | | | ▢ |
| W5 | 176 | 124 | Night Sky | 8–10 | U | | ✓ | | | |
| W5 | 177 | 127 | Personal Vitality Kit | 5 | U | | ✂ | | | |
| W5 | 178 | 129 | Sights for Sore Eyes | 1–2 | U | | | | | |
| W5 | 179 | 132 | Stimulate and Integrate | 4–5 | U | | | | | |
| W5 | 180 | 134 | Strike Three | 3 | U | | | | | |

KEY on page 2

| CATEGORY | EXERCISE # | WORKSITE | FAVORITES | INTRODUCTIONS | CHALKTALK | DEMO | RELAXATION | SCRIPT | ACTIVITY | SMALL GROUPS | LARGE GROUP | DISCLOSURE | TRAINER PREP |
|---|---|---|---|---|---|---|---|---|---|---|---|---|---|
| **Wellness 3** | | | | | | | | | | | | | |
| | 106 | ♦ | | | | ➤ | | | | | ✳ | ❷ | |
| | 107 | | | | | ➤ | ♦ | | ♦ | ✛ | | | |
| | 108 | | | | | ➤ | ♦ | 99 | ♦ | ✛ | | | |
| **Wellness 4** | | | | | | | | | | | | | |
| | 135 | | | | | | ♦ | | ♦ | | | | ❶ |
| | 136 | | | | | | ♦ | | ♦ | | | | |
| | 137 | | | | | | ♦ | 99 | ♦ | | | | |
| | 138 | | | | | | | 99 | ♦ | | | | ❷ |
| | 139 | | | | | | | 99 | | | | | |
| | 140 | | | | ● | | | | | ✛ | ✳ | | |
| | 141 | ♦ | | | | | | 99 | | | | | |
| | 142 | | | | ● | ➤ | | | ♦ | | ✳ | | |
| | 143 | | | | | ➤ | ♦ | 99 | | | ✳ | | ❶ |
| | 144 | ♦ | | | | | | | | | ✳ | | |
| **Wellness 5** | | | | | | | | | | | | | |
| | 171 | ♦ | | | | | | | | | | | ❶ |
| | 172 | | | | ● | ➤ | ♦ | 99 | | | | | |
| | 173 | | ☆ | | ● | ➤ | | | ♦ | | | | ❶ |
| | 174 | | ☆ | | | | | | | | | | ❶ |
| | 175 | ♦ | | | | | | | | ✛ | ✳ | | ❶ |
| | 176 | | | | | | ♦ | 99 | | | | | |
| | 177 | ♦ | | | | ➤ | | | ♦ | | | | ❸ |
| | 178 | ♦ | | | | ➤ | ♦ | 99 | ♦ | | | | |
| | 179 | | | | ● | ➤ | | 99 | ♦ | | | | |
| | 180 | ♦ | ☆ | | | | | 99 | | | | | |

KEY on page 2

©1995 Whole Person Press 210 W Michigan Duluth MN 55802 (800) 247-6789

# 2
# Annotated Indexes

If you are looking for specific content material or thematic group experiences, check out these *Annotated Indexes* which briefly summarize the content and process of lecturettes (called *chalktalks*), demonstrations, mental and physical energizers, and relaxation routines in the ten volumes of the series, with appropriate page numbers for easy reference.

© 1995  Whole Person Press 210 W Michigan Duluth MN 55802      (800) 247-6789

## STRESS 2            PAGE                     CHALKTALKS

## STRESS 3         PAGE                             CHALKTALKS

© 1995  Whole Person Press 210 W Michigan Duluth MN 55802      (800) 247-6789

**STRESS 5**                    PAGE                          **CHALKTALKS**

© 1995  Whole Person Press 210 W Michigan Duluth MN 55802        (800) 247-6789

## WELLNESS 2      PAGE              CHALKTALKS

© 1995  Whole Person Press 210 W Michigan Duluth MN 55802     (800) 247-6789

## WELLNESS 3        PAGE                 CHALKTALKS

© 1995  Whole Person Press 210 W Michigan Duluth MN 55802        (800) 247-6789

© 1995 Whole Person Press 210 W Michigan Duluth MN 55802       (800) 247-6789

| STRESS 4 | PAGE | DEMONSTRATIONS |
|---|---|---|
| 116 Body Mapping | 21 | Consciousness-raising process with a nice chalk-talk on physical consequences of stress. |
| 129 Biofeedback | 92 | Use Biodots to demonstrate the effects of relaxation. Includes the *I am Relaxed* autogenic script. Nice chalktalk on biofeedback and the stress/relaxation response. |
| 138 Human Knots | 120 | Groups of 6–20 people tie themselves in knots to demonstrate the physical effects of stress, then untangle again to experience the benefits of relaxation. |
| 139 Merry-Go-Round | 122 | Participants simulate the stress of taking on too many burdens as they juggle an increasing number of objects. |

| STRESS 5 | PAGE | DEMONSTRATIONS |
|---|---|---|
| 150 Ton of Bricks | 14 | A brick serves as a metaphor for the weight of life stresses. |
| 159 Stress Management Alphabet | 60 | Cross-patterning exercise for right and left brain balance. |
| | 61 | Participants make an on-the-spot commitment to participate in an invigorating group backrub. |
| | 62 | Stretching and visualization routine that challenges participants to do something different. |
| | 63 | The skill of exaggeration is demonstrated with handshakes. |
| 163 Keep Your Cool | 87 | Short role play of skills for anger management. |
| | 87 | *In vivo* practice of skills for handling provocative situations. |
| 164 Remote Control | 91 | Vivid demonstration of making choices about our actions and attitudes. |
| | 92 | Participants explore their natural power to change their feelings by changing their thoughts. |
| 165 Yoga | 95 | The relaxing effects of yoga breathing techniques. |
| | 97 | Assume the basic relaxation posture of yoga. |
| 173 Cobra | 118 | Gentle yoga movements for stretching the back and stimulating inner organs. |
| 177 Superman | 126 | Graphic illustration of human imperfection. |

© 1995  Whole Person Press 210 W Michigan Duluth MN 55802        (800) 247-6789

**103 Balancing Act**     123 Pairs demonstrate the dynamic process of maintaining a healthy balance.

**108 Weather Report**    132 Participants practice techniques to release muscle tension in their partner's neck, shoulders, and back.

| WELLNESS 4 | PAGE | DEMONSTRATIONS |
|---|---|---|

**116 Whole Person Potpourri**     23 Participants demonstrate whole person well-being concepts using intriguing tools and models.

**117 Health and Lifestyle**     34 Be sure to stop the film and guide the group in an experience of Herbert Benson's classic *relaxation response.*

**119 Symphony of the Cells**     46 Groups dramatically demonstrate the components and functions of physical and nonphysical human systems.

**121 Take a Walk!**     52 Monitoring heart rate before, during, and after exercise.

**142 On Purpose**     127 This demonstration highlights the importance of intentionality and concentration in healthy lifestyle choice and developing new habits.

**143 Sensory Relaxation**     129 Excellent demonstration of the power of sensory awareness.

| WELLNESS 5 | PAGE | DEMONSTRATIONS |
|---|---|---|

**150 Family Health Tree**     17 Demonstrates how to understand a genogram and use it as a tool for exploring family history.

**162 Seven Ways of Knowing**     77 On the spot IQ test demonstrates seven intelligent approaches to problem solving.

**172 Cleansing Breath**     115 Basic yoga alternate side breathing technique.

**173 For the Health of It**     118 Lively dance steps are taught by the trainer and enjoyed by participants.

**178 Sights for Sore Eyes**     130 Trainer shows participants how to treat themselves to a revitalizing "bath" for tired eyes.

**179 Stimulate and Integrate**     132 Step-by-step instructions for do-it-yourself sensory integration.

© 1995 Whole Person Press 210 W Michigan Duluth MN 55802 (800) 247-6789

| **WELLNESS 2** | PAGE | **PHYSICAL ENERGIZERS** |
|---|---|---|

| **WELLNESS 3** | PAGE | **PHYSICAL ENERGIZERS** |
|---|---|---|

© 1995  Whole Person Press 210 W Michigan Duluth MN 55802        (800) 247-6789

© 1995  Whole Person Press 210 W Michigan Duluth MN 55802        (800) 247-6789

## WELLNESS 1           PAGE                    MENTAL ENERGIZERS

© 1995  Whole Person Press 210 W Michigan Duluth MN 55802        (800) 247-6789

© 1995  Whole Person Press 210 W Michigan Duluth MN 55802        (800) 247-6789

© 1995 Whole Person Press 210 W Michigan Duluth MN 55802          (800) 247-6789

© 1995  Whole Person Press 210 W Michigan Duluth MN 55802        (800) 247-6789

# 3
# Winning
# Combinations

The *Winning Combinations* section includes thirty stress and wellness presentation/workshop outlines, ranging from 45 minutes to a full day to several weekly sessions—all using combinations of structured exercises from one or more volumes in the series. Whether you are planning an evening presentation for a community group, developing a course for your workplace, or designing an education group for clients/patients/students, use these outlines as a springboard for your own creativity.

## WINNING COMBINATIONS                                       STRESS 1

### ▓ One-Shot Stress and Coping Presentation        (10–60 min)

For a brief (10–20 minute) presentation, use the process described in *Stress Risk Factors* (S1.10, 10–20 min).

For a longer time slot (30–50 minutes), try *The Juggling Act* (S1.8, 40–60 min) *or Personal Stressors and Copers* (S1.6, 20–30 min). Both include stress assessment segments as well as strategies for coping.

For a memorable hour-long presentation, use the extended *Juggling Act* process, or the complete version of *The AAAbc's of Stress Management* (S1.12, 45–60 min).

### ▓ Half-Day Workshop Focusing on Coping            (2–3 hours)

Begin the workshop with a focused group warm-up, using *Rummage Sale* (S1.1c, 15–20 min) or *Stress Symptom Inventory* (S1.7, 30–40 min). The latter process can be shortened effectively to a 10–15 minute icebreaker if you drop the drawing and sharing sections, *Steps 4* and *6*.

The major portion of the workshop focuses on stress assessment using *The Juggling Act* (S1.8, 40–60 min) followed by an exploration of management strategies via *Coping Skills Assessment* (S1.14, 45–60 min).

Close the workshop with the systematic planning process in *One Step at a Time* (S1.22, 20–30 min).

### ▓ Full-Day Workshop Focusing on Coping            (5–6 hours)

Follow the sequence for the half-day workshop, using the extended process for each exercise. Insert *Skill Skits* (S1.15, 60 min) after the *Coping Skills Assessment*. Substitute the closing *Postscript* (S1.23, 15 min) for *One Step at a Time*.

### ▓ Workaholism Workshop                            (1–3 hours)

Although current research suggests that the relationship between the *Type A* personality and heart disease may not be as valid as Rosenman and Friedman first hypothesized, nearly everyone agrees that the workaholic lifestyle is stressful.

*Lifetrap 1:Workaholism* (S1.11, 60–90 min) provides an extended stress and lifestyle exploration that helps participants consider the meaning of work in their lives and uncover the belief system that drives them. This topic seems to have universal appeal. To expand or spice up your presentation, try adding one or more of the following "natural companions."

◆ Harried *Type As* usually have lots on their minds. Help them take a mental stress break with *Clear the Deck!* (S1.3, 10–15 min).

◆ The worksheet (*Steps 2* and *3*) from *The Juggling Act* (S1.8, 10 min) is a nice warm-up for the over-stressed.

◆ Use the statements from the *Workaholic Belief Systems* worksheet (p. 47 in *Stress 1*) as the litany for *Boo-Down* (S1.25, 5–8 min).

◆ *Type As* are often unaware of their tension level. The demonstration in *Tension Hurts* (S1.36, 5 min) helps people get in touch with tension.

◆ Use *Slow Me Down Lord* (S1.18c, 3 min) for a serious, thought-provoking ending. Try the "Type A Theme Song" from *Singalong 2* (S1.32, 3 min) for a rousing closure.

© 1995 Whole Person Press 210 W Michigan Duluth MN 55802        (800) 247-6789

If you have other volumes in the *Structured Exercises* series, you can add even more pizzazz to your workshop:

◆ Substitute *Turtle, Hare or Racehorse?* (S2.38, 20–30 min) for the *Type A—Type B* continuum in *Step 3,* or combine the processes.

◆ Use *Month of Fundays* (S2.50, 20–30 min) to insert playfulness as part of your presentation on coping skills.

◆ The delightful parable on play, *The Garden* (S2.63, 5 min), is particularly applicable to the workaholic.

◆ Another parable, *What's the Hurry?* (S3.106, 5 min), poignantly highlights the ultimate consequences of the hurry sickness, and could be used effectively as an introduction, illustration, or wrap-up to your workshop.

## WINNING COMBINATIONS                                         STRESS 2

### ▓ One-Shot Stress Management Presentation          (10–90 min)

For a short (10–20 min) presentation, use the process described in *Circuit Overload* (S2.47, 15–20 min) or a brief version of *The Worry Stopper* (S2.51, 30–40 min).

For a longer time slot (30–50 min), try *The Fourth Source of Stress* (S2.42, 45–60 min) or *Dragnet* (S2.44, 30–40 min). Use an appropriate icebreaker from *Introductions 4* (S2.37, 10–20 min) and add *Four Quadrant Questions* (S2.39, 10–15 min) for closure.

For a memorable, hour-long presentation, begin by using *Circuit Overload* (S2.47, 15–20 min). Then focus on personal management styles with *PILEUP Copers* (S2.49, 45–60 min).

### ▓ Workshop on Stress and Self-Esteem          (90 min–3 hours)

Begin with *Life Event Bingo* (S2.40, 10–20 min). This mixer based on Holmes and Rahe's Social Readjustment Rating Scale highlights life changes that may be stressful.

The major portion of the workshop focuses on four sources of stress: anticipated life events, unexpected life events, accumulated strains, and personal trait stress (self-esteem). Use *The Fourth Source of Stress* (S2.42, 45–60 min), expanding your presentation of the first three sources as described on p. 18. Then spend the major portion of time exploring self-esteem as a stress generator and stress reliever.

For a longer session or workshop, incorporate an esteem-building, skill-training component here. Use *Speak Up!* (S2.54, 40–45 min) to focus on assertiveness skills, or try *Affirmative Action Plan* (S2.55, 40–50 min), using oneself (rather than a co-worker) as the target.

Be sure to allow time for one of these affirming closures to the learning experience:
*PILEUP Copers* (S2.49, 60 min)
*Manager of the Year* (S2.59, 45–60 min)
*Treasure Chest* (S2.72, 15–20 min)

### ▓ Hooked on Helping Workshop          (90 min–3 hours)

For years we conducted two-day workshops focused on the special stresses of the helping professions. The process described in *Lifetrap 2: Hooked on Helping* (S2.46, 60–90 min) is the heart of that workshop. Even if your audience is not exclusively health care or social service personnel, nearly everyone can identify with the issues of over-extension on the job and/or in relationships.

To expand your presentation of this important stress issue, choose one or more of the following "natural companions" from *Stress 2.*

◆ The icebreaker *Wave the Magic Wand* (S2.37c, 2–4 min) may help helpers articulate their unrealistic expectations and hopes for a magical solution.

◆ The format of *Exclusive Interview* (S2.41, 25–30 min) appeals to human service professionals—they usually have good interviewing skills and enjoy the self-discovery process. Good starting point—or recast the questions to use as a closing assessment.

◆ Job burnout is a critical issue for helpers. Incorporate *Burnout Index* (S2.43, 10–15 min) into your exploration of the addiction trap in *Part C.*

◆ *Back to the Drawing Board* (S2.45, 50–75 min) makes a great companion exercise for a longer workshop format.

◆ Play is a natural remedy for over-stressed care-givers. Include *Month of Fundays* (S2.50, 20–30 min) as a skill-builder.

◆ Most helpers have difficulty saying NO and asking for what they need. *Speak Up!* (S2.54, 40–45 min) is a perfect skill-building module for an extended learning experience.

◆ Be sure to read *The Garden* (S2.63, 5 min) sometime during your presentation. It's a perfect parable for the over-burdened.

◆ *Hand-to-Hand Contact* (S2.64, 10 min) allows participants to practice receiving as well as giving.

◆ For a nice closing visualization try *Treasure Chest* (S2.72, 15–20 min). Participants discover a "gift" they need.

If you have other volumes in the *Structured Exercises* series, you can add even more pizzazz to your workshop:

◆ Try the checklist from *Stress Symptom Inventory* (S1.7, 10–40 min) as an introduction to *Hooked on Helping.* Should help people get in touch with the cost of caring.

◆ The process in *Obligation Overload* (S4.122, 45 min) provides an effective skill session for the overburdened.

◆ Don't miss *Merry-Go-Round* (S4.139, 5–15 min)—a rowdy demonstration of the stress of taking on too many burdens.

## WINNING COMBINATIONS                                                    STRESS 3

### ▧ Generic Stress Presentation                                         (60–90 min)

Start with the chalktalk and stress thermometer warm-up in *Spice or Arsenic?* (S3.79, 20–30 min) which helps people focus on their current, past, and target stress level.

Then introduce the overarching paradigm for coping with stress outlined in *S.O.S. for Stress* (S3.86, 30–50 min). As you present the three strategies: Start on the Situation, Start on Self, and Seek out Support, throw in some energizers to illustrate the strategies and give the group a break.

© 1995 Whole Person Press 210 W Michigan Duluth MN 55802          (800) 247-6789

Close your workshop with the powerfully motivating visualization/goal-setting process in *Imagine Success* (S3.89, 15–30 min).

## ▓ Workshop on Stress with Skill-Building Component (Listening or Conflict Management)                    (2 hours)

When stress management is the topic of a class or workshop, trainers (and participants!) often spend more time on stress than on management. If you'd like to help a group focus on coping, build an entire workshop around one of the two major stress management skills appropriate in nearly any setting: listening and managing conflict.

Begin either workshop with *Traveling Trios* (S3.77, 10–15 min). This lively icebreaker helps people get acquainted (or reacquainted) as they compare coping styles. If you'd like a more didactic warm-up, try substituting *S.O.S. for Stress* (S3.86, 30–50 min) as a good, basic introduction to stress management strategies.

◆ For a **listening skills** focus, introduce the subject with the powerful demonstration *You're Not Listening!* (S3.107, 5–10 min). Then, to teach effective listening skills in triads, use *Stop Look and Listen* (S3.92, 60 min).

◆ For a **conflict management** focus, use the thought-provoking demonstration in *Tug of War* (S3.104, 5–10 min) to help people analyze their typical reactions to conflict. Then teach the four skills for dealing with conflict as presented in *Conflict Management* (S3.90, 60 min) and allow participants to apply the strategies to specific conflict situations in their lives.

*Exit Interview* (S3.95, 20–30 min) combines closure with skill practice. Use it with either the **listening** or **conflict** workshop to reinforce the stress management skills that you've presented.

## ▓ Stress and Change Workshop                         (90 min–3 hours)

*Lifetrap 3: Sick of Change* (S3.82, 60–90 min) uses the most famous stress assessment, Holmes and Rahe's Social Readjustment Rating Scale as the centerpiece for exploring the role of change in our lives and the stress it creates. All audiences should be able to identify with the issues and appreciate the focus on strategies for managing change. To expand or spice up your presentation, try adding one or more of these "natural companions."

◆ The stress thermometer in *Spice or Arsenic?* (S3.79, 20–30 min) makes a nice additional warm-up to the topic of change.

◆ Expand *Part B* to include *Stress Clusters Clinic* (S3.87, 40–60 min). This exercise, using PILEUP cards, graphically demonstrates the stress of accumulated life changes and creative options for dealing with it.

◆ Use the visualization in *Imagine Success* (S3.89, 15–30 min) to reinforce the planning process, or try *Recipe for Success with Stress* (S3.96, 25–30 min) after the planning and sharing process. Invite participants to read their recipes out loud.

Don't forget to change the rhythm of your workshop with tension-relieving breaks and creative activities. This volume contains several excellent energizers and demonstrations. Pick one or more that tickle your fancy.

◆ Sprinkle several energizers from *Eight-Minute Stress Break* (S3.91, 1 min each) throughout your presentation for a change of pace. Or have some fun as you kick up your heels with *Kicking Your Stress Can-Can* (S3.99, 5 min).

◆ Try *Chinese Swing* (S3.100, 10 min) as a healthy midsession break. This technique practiced regularly can be a powerful antidote to the stress of change. *Clouds to Sunshine* (S3.101, 3–5 min) teaches a simple yoga stretch as it demonstrates that change is as inevitable as the seasons.

◆ Creativity, camaraderie, and reinforcement of key concepts are natural outcomes of *Create a Singalong* (S3.102, 10–15 min), when small groups make up songs about stress and change.

If you have lots of time you might want to add one of these effective warm-ups from other volumes in the series before *Part A*.

◆ *Life Event Bingo* (S2.40, 10–20 min) was designed specifically to introduce the concepts of Holmes and Rahe's scale while people get acquainted.

◆ *Stress Symptom Inventory* (S1.7, 30–40 min) provides a whole person assessment that really helps people get in touch with the manifestations of stress in their life.

## WINNING COMBINATIONS                                    STRESS 4

### ▒ Job Stress Presentation                                    (60 min)

Begin your workshop with a topical icebreaker. *Quips and Quotes* (S4.111, 20–30 min) can be shortened to 10 minutes by using only *Steps 1* and *2* as an icebreaker. Participants choose catchy slogans that typify their approach to stress management. Or shorten *Stress Attitudes Survey* (S4.118, 20–30 min) to 10 minutes by choosing 2–3 statements for a quick warm-up vote (*Steps 1–3*). Then pick one statement particularly appropriate to your audience and setting for brief small group discussions.

Use *On the Job Stress Grid* (S4.117, 25–40 min) as the centerpiece of your presentation. Participants brainstorm sources of job stress, then use two worksheets to pinpoint their personal job "hot spots." The *Job Stress Grid* is a great tool for exploring workplace stressors. Expand the closing chalktalk on coping strategies to make a smooth transition to planning. Drop the homework.

Sometime during the session participants will mention difficult co-workers or a hostile work environment as sources of stress. When this issue comes up, stop and share the reading in *How to Swim with Sharks* (S4.137, 5 min). It's a real gem.

Close your presentation with an effective planning process. *So What?* (S4.131, 10–15 min) is simple, satisfying, and memorable. Or incorporate *ABCDEFG Planner* (S4.130, 20–30 min) as a natural extension of the *Job Stress Grid*. Use the "hot spot" generated in *Step 7* of the *Grid* as the "problem" in *Section A* of the *Planner*. Use the three "options for coping with organizational stress" from *Step 8* as strategies for *Section E* of the *Planner*.

If you have time, add one or more energizers. *Giraffe* (S4.135, 5 min) provides a quick stretch. *Sigh of Relief* (S4.143, 3–5 min) is an easy but powerful stress reliever. *Snap, Crackle, Pop* (S4.144, 5 min) is a lively three-person back massage that peps up a group.

### ▒ Focus on the Physical: Stress and Relaxation          (90 min)

*Dear Me* (S4.113, 10–15 min) makes a nice reflective opening. Follow up with the life-size stress assessment in *Body Mapping* (S4.116, 30–45 min). Participants scan

---

© 1995 Whole Person Press 210 W Michigan Duluth MN 55802          (800) 247-6789

their bodies for tension, then pair up to map physical stress. Supplement the chalktalk with more information on the physical stress reaction and our inclination to ignore or override it.

Introduce the basic principles of relaxation as an antidote to stress using *Biofeedback* (S4.129, 20–25 min). Miniature thermometers (Biodots) help people monitor fluctuating stress levels as they practice a simple relaxation routine. Again, beef up the opening chalktalk on the relaxation response.

Choose several additional relaxation routines to demonstrate the variety of tension-relievers available. This volume includes several: *Giraffe* (S4.135, 5 min), *Hot Tub* (S4.136, 8 min), *Human Knots* (S4.138, 5–10 min), *Microwave* (S4.140, 2 min), *Revitalize Your Eyes* (S4.142, 2–5 min each), *Sigh of Relief* (S4.143, 3–5 min), *Snap, Crackle, Pop* (S4.144, 5–10 min). Or check the *Annotated Indexes,* p. 35, for more information.

To close the session, use the companion process to your opening. *Dear Me P.S.* (S4.134, 10–15 min) gives participants an opportunity to evaluate what they have learned and apply it to personal life situations.

### ▒ Good Grief Workshop                                  (1.5– 2.5 hours)
Grief is a universal human experience—and a major source of stress and illness. Whether the loss is the death of a parent or a corporate restructuring, we are all vulnerable to the stressful lifetrap of saying "goodbye." Although this subject may seem too "personal" for intact groups in the work setting, we think the prevalence of relationships as "high stress" issues and the demonstrated correlation between grief and physical illness may make it worth the risk to explore this topic as an entry point to stress management.

*Lifetrap 4: Good Grief* (S4.120, 60–90 min) provides an excellent structure for addressing the stress of letting go. This exercise assumes that the group has a general background knowledge about stress. If not, be sure to add some generic stress information to the opening chalktalk. To extend the process or to include a more in-depth coping skill presentation and practice, try these "natural companions."

◆ Use *Barometer* (S4.109b, 5–10 min, 1 min per person—divide into groups of 4–8) as an icebreaker. This quick introduction helps people focus on their recent life experience.

◆ Be sure to read the *Mustard Seed* parable (S4.141, 5 min) after your opening chalktalk. It's an absolute classic.

◆ Follow up your "closing" chalktalk with an exploration of self-disclosure as an appropriate skill for coping with grief using *Open Up* (S4.128, 30–40 min). The list of "helping" resources generated by the group may be especially valuable.

◆ A closing planning/implementation process will promote better transfer of learning. Try *911 Emergency Plan* (S4.124, 20-30 min), an outstanding exercise for developing a personalized plan for managing crisis situations so common to grief reactions. Or substitute *So What?* (S4.131, 10–15 min) or *Dear Me P.S.* (S4.134, 10–15 min) as described above.

## WINNING COMBINATIONS                                                 STRESS 5

### ▓ Coping with Stress: Managing Anger and Anxiety          (1-2 hours)

For most people, anger and anxiety are typical stress responses—and frequent stress escalators. A skill-building workshop geared to help people manage these feelings would be appropriate for nearly any audience or setting.

Begin with a mood-setting warm-up, *One-Minute Autobiographies* (S5.148, 10–20 min). Direct folks to tell their life stories by focusing on episodes of anger or anxiety only.

*Keep Your Cool* (S5.163, 60–90 min) vividly demonstrates how we can be directors rather than victims of our feelings. Although the exercise is geared toward managing anger, the process and content apply equally well to anxiety. You could choose to focus on one of these problems or combine both in a single session. Adapt the role play scenarios to generate the desired feeling(s). If time is limited, reduce the number of scenarios.

◆ Be sure to include *Remote Control* (S5.164, 20–30 min). This vivid demonstration of people's power to regulate their moods and actions in unforgettable.

◆ If you have time, use the visualization in *Trouble Bubbles* (S5.179, 5–10 min) as an additional demonstration of controlling anger or anxiety by relaxing and blowing away the negative feelings.

For an uplifting ending, try *Go Fly a Kite* (S5.167, 10–20 min). Modify the questions to focus on the stress of anxiety or anger. Encourage everyone to create a plan for managing these feelings that is guaranteed to fly.

As a farewell ritual, create *Stress Squeezers* (S5.176, 10–15 min) and encourage people to use these flexible toys as tools for releasing anxiety and anger by squeezing them whenever they start to feel stressed out.

### ▓ Workshop on the Hardiness Factor                            (2-3 hours)

If you're tired of Selye's eustress/distress theory, *Type A* behavior, and the stress of Life Change Events, try a presentation or workshop that focuses on assessing and building stress resistance.

Start the workshop with a short group warm-up using *Nametag Questions* (S5.147, 15–20 min), tailoring the questions to hardiness issues. Modify the time as needed by varying the number of times people change partners.

The chalktalks and assessment in *The Hardiness Factor* (S5.151, 30–40 min) provide a broad introduction to Kobasa's research on stress resistance and specific feedback to participants on their relative strength in the three hardiness traits: challenge, commitment, and control.

◆ **Challenge**. *Silver Linings* (S5.158, 20–30 min) is perfect for discovering opportunities (challenge) in stressful situations.

◆ **Commitment**. To expand on this topic use *Life and Death Questions* (W2.56, 20–30 min with group sharing omitted) or *Expanding Your Circles* (W4.125, 20–30 min).

◆ **Control**. *Pick Your Battles* (S5.153, 30 min) or *Yesterday, Today, and Tomorrow* (S5.160, 20–30 min) address issues of control in stress management.

© 1995 Whole Person Press 210 W Michigan Duluth MN 55802          (800) 247-6789

*Try, Try Again* (S5.180, 5 min) or *Hand Dancing* (S5.174, 10 min) provide playful energizers dealing with control and letting go.

◆ The concept of physical resilience can be introduced by *Yoga* (S5.165, 30–60 min), *Cobra* (S5.173, 5 min), or *Humming Breath* (S5.175, 3–5 min).

For planning and closure, *Key Learning* (S5.169, 5–10 min) is well-suited. If you have other volumes of the *Structured Exercises* series, you can add more pizzazz to your workshop by substituting *Stress Buffer Shield* (S1.16, 20–30 min).

## ▧ Superwoman Stress Workshop                                    (2–4 hours)

Women comprise the largest segment of audiences at stress management programs. If you'd like to address the special issues women face, build a workshop around *Lifetrap 5: Superwoman Syndrome* (S5.152, 60–90 min).

Begin with *Badge of My Profession* (S5.146, 15–20 min), adapting the worksheet questions to fit the role of Superwomen. Then proceed through the analysis of *Superwoman* stress: myths, stress symptoms, guilt and expectations, entitlement, and strategies for change. Since low self-esteem is a chronic issue for so many women, incorporate *Affirmation Calendar* (S5.161, 25–30 min) as a part of *Step 13*.

To expand the skill-building focus of your workshop, include *Eating Under Stress* (S5.162, 40–45 min) or *Yoga* (S5.165, 30–60 min), which are both superb skills for Superwomen.

Conclude with an affirming female systems process for gathering insights and resolutions: *Hope Chest* (S5.168, 15–20 min).

Be sure to take frequent breaks—Superwomen tend to ignore their self-care needs.

◆ *Superman* (S5.177, 5–10 min) is sure to get a laugh.

◆ *Humming Breath* (S5.175, 3–5 min) and *Breath Prayer* (S5.172, 8–10 min) are powerful energizers.

◆ If you have time, insert *Mealtime Meditation* (W5.157, 10–15 min) before a lunch break.

## WINNING COMBINATIONS                                              WELLNESS 1

## ▧ Whole Person Wellness and Self-Care                        (50–75 min)

*Whole Person Health Appraisal* (W1.6, 20–30 min) provides a good introduction to the broad, whole person view of wellness, and challenges people to assess their self-care practices and identify their personal risk factors in six dimensions of wellness: physical, mental, emotional, social, spiritual, and lifestyle. Follow this assessment process with the powerful self-care metaphor, *The Marathon Strategy* (W1.11, 15 min).

Close with the whole person *Real to Ideal* (W1.24, 10–15 min) planner, or *What Do You Need?* (W1.23, 10–15 min). Stop along the way for a *Group Backrub* (W1.31, 2–5 min), some *60-Second Tension Tamers* (W1.27, 1 min each), or a *Singalong* (W1.35, 2–5 min).

If you have a longer time, begin with the icebreaker, *Ten Qualities of the Super Well,* (W1.5, 25–30 min), which engages participants in an intense discussion of their concepts about health as well as their personal priorities and biases. Or try *Wellness Goals/Health Concerns* (W1.1c, 5–10 min). Then add one or more body/mind/spirit self-care processes after the marathon image.

If you have plenty of time and are working with a work team or another group that will be spending time together in the future, you might want to include *Wellness Congress* (W1.9, 90–120 min). This process builds group camaraderie as everyone works toward consensus in developing a wellness creed.

## ▓ Mini-Workshop on
## Health/Illness Patterns and Self-Responsibility          (2 hours)

Insurance companies and employers who fund health benefits for their employees are particularly interested in the cost containment potential of wellness programs that focus on what the individual can do to prevent future diseases. This volume has several exercises that cultivate this dynamic of self-responsibility.

Begin the mini-workshop with the *Two-Minute Mill* (W1.2, 10–15 min), selecting conversation topics that provoke discussion about concepts of wellness, health or illness patterns of the past, self-care habits, etc. If you have time, invite the participants to assess their current health status in a group with the *Human Health/ Illness Continuum* (W1.3, 10–20 min).

The major learning of the session will come through the introspective journey outlined in *Health/Illness Images* (W1.10, 90 min). This extended reflection exercise helps participants recognize the ebb and flow of sickness and health in their lives and often prompts a dramatic perceptual shift to a sharper sense of self-responsibility.

Be sure to read the *Grabwell Grommet* story (W1.30, 5 min) sometime during the workshop. It can be a great opening attention getter, a natural transition between processes, or a powerful wrap-up. You also might want to include a few short self-care breaks from the group energizers.

Wind up the workshop with the open-ended *Shoulds, Wants, Wills* (W1.22, 15–20 min), or another self-care planner of your choice.

## ▓ Warm-Up to Wellness Kickoff          (1–2 hours)

This design is for an introductory session of a multipart wellness course or long workshop. The goal is to explore the meaning of wellness and develop a shared conceptual framework to build on for future assessment and self-care sessions.

Begin with an icebreaker from *Introductions 1* (W1.1, 5–10 min). *Analogies* or *Jingles* would work well. If possible, take time for the *Wellness Congress* (W1.9, 90–120 min), which will help the group warm up to wellness concepts and build group spirit. If you are pressed for time, at least do the section on writing a group *Wellness Creed*.

Once the group has generated a vision of what might be possible with high level wellness, invite participants to assess their present well-being and identify areas for potential healthy changes. *Whole Person Health Appraisal* (W1.6, 20–30) works well, or choose from the many exploration/appraisal tools in other volumes in this series.

You may want to conduct a plenary session following this process and solicit from the group their needs, hopes, and expectations for the learning experience. This feedback will help you choose appropriate exercises for the remaining sessions.

Close with an adaptation of *Meet the New Me* (W1.26, 10–15 min), where participants introduce themselves as if they had accomplished the goals they have set for the course/workshop.

© 1995 Whole Person Press 210 W Michigan Duluth MN 55802          (800) 247-6789

During a long workshop it is especially important to include periodic group energizers that fit the content of what you are presenting. You might want to use *Red Rover* (W1.34, 5–15 min) during this initial session to demonstrate through analogy that people *can* live life differently.

Homework can be a very effective learning tool. Invite participants to try the *Noontime Energizers* (W1.33, 5–10 min) assignment at several points between sessions, keeping track of their experiences in a journal or log. At the next session, spend a few minutes sharing insights from these journals in dyads or small groups before launching into the next content area.

## WINNING COMBINATIONS                                    WELLNESS 2

### ▨ Whole Person Wellness Presentation              (70–90 minutes)

If you have only one opportunity to impact a group on wellness issues, we recommend that you start with the basics. Provide an opportunity to explore the concept of wellness from a whole person perspective that looks at symptoms of dis-ease, possible causes of ill-health, treatment options, and signs of health in five dimensions of being: physical, emotional, spiritual, relational, and intellectual.

Begin with the icebreaker *"Quality Circles"* (W2.38, 10–15 min). Participants choose from an array of whole person well-being characteristics and use this "quality" to introduce themselves.

The heart of the presentation follows *Wheel of Health* (W2.46, 60–90 min), the process Don developed to teach the whole person concept to patients and providers for the Wholistic Health Centers project nationwide. You can easily condense the demonstration in *Part B* and use dyads instead of large group discussion in *Part C* if your time is short.

If you plan a break during your presentation, you could convert this "dead" time to productive interaction if you assign an appropriate brainstorming or discussion task as described in *Working Coffee Break* (W2.71, 5–10 min). Ask people to pair up and talk about typical symptom areas or preferred treatment choices or their favorite wellness signs.

If this session is a kick-off for a longer course, poll the audience at the conclusion of the *Wheel* exercise to determine which areas of well-being they would like to consider in more depth in future sessions.

### ▨ Wellness and Meaning in Life Presentation          (1–2 hours)

The heart of this presentation is the *Caring Appraisal* (W2.44, 45–60 min). This alternative exploration of whole person well-being begins with an inventory of health habits and self-care practices in four dimensions: physical, mental, relational, and spiritual, plus an appraisal of the ways that they reach out to care for others from their position of well-being.

If you have time, follow up with the powerful *Life and Death Questions* (W2.56, 30–60 min), participants will have an opportunity to affirm their values and beliefs as they clarify personal goals for well-being.

With a conservative audience, try the opening/closing pair *Roundup* (W2.37a, 5–15 min) and *Roundup Revisited* (W2.59, 1–2 min per person). If your group is more adventurous, use *Pocket or Purse* (W2.37c, 5–15 min) as an icebreaker and *Vital Signs* (W2.62, 10–15 min) for closure.

### ■ Self-Care Presentation, Workshop, or Course        (1–8 hours)

Use any of the *Introductions 3* (W2.37, 5–15 min) icebreakers as a warm-up. Then move on to a process that will help participants identify self-care goals by evaluating their *(My) Present Health Status* (W2.43, 30–40 min). After the small group sharing in *Step 6,* reconvene the entire group to identify self-care issues people would like to work on further.

◆ The *One-A-Day Plan* (W2.61, 10–30 min) provides a nice generic strategy for setting a month's worth of self-care goals for one or several issues.

If this is the first session of a multipart course, you can plan a tentative agenda for upcoming sessions based on the expressed needs of the group. See the list below for some suggestions.

If this is the first part of a half-day or daylong workshop, you should come prepared with three or four processes dealing with self-care issues you anticipate the group will choose. Where you can, correlate the identified concerns with the self-care processes you have prepared. If the audience is hot for a topic you're not prepared for, acknowledge the fact that those needs probably won't be met directly during this workshop, but be ready to suggest some alternative strategies for learning.

If you've anticipated well, participants' feedback should provide a natural transition to your next self-care agenda. *Wellness 2* includes several intriguing exercises for addressing a variety of self-care issues:

◆ *Self-Care Learning Contract* (W2.47, 5–10 min) and *Wish List* (W2.48, 5 min each session) help people focus on progress towards goals.

◆ *Annual Physical* (W2.49, 30–45 min), *Personal Fitness Check* (W2.51, 60 min), and *Medicine Cabinet* (W2.52, 45–60 min) explore different aspects of physical self-care. And don't miss the opportunity to incorporate the astonishing eating habits experience in *Lunch Duets* (W2.50, 1–2 hours).

◆ *Loneliness Locator* (W2.54, 60–90) takes a look at an important mental health/ interpersonal issue. *Compass* (W2.55, 30–60 min) and *Life and Death Questions* (W2.56, 30–60 min) provide an opportunity to tap into the internal wisdom of the spirit dimension, looking for balance, purpose, and motivation for lifestyle questions.

◆ The unusual *Self-Care SOAP* assessment (W2.57, 90 min) can be used to look at any physical or whole person symptom configuration in more detail.

See p. 141 for suggested self-care energizers *Especially for the Workplace*—or nearly any setting.

## WINNING COMBINATIONS                                    WELLNESS 3

### ■ Whole Person Wellness Presentation Plus      (45–90 minutes)

*Personal Wellness Wheel* (W3.79, 15–20 min) is an excellent centerpiece for any wellness presentation. The eight dimensions of well-being allow for affirmation as well as confrontation about wellness patterns and areas of concern.

Follow up this general assessment with one or more thematic self-care processes that you anticipate will be important to your audience.

© 1995 Whole Person Press 210 W Michigan Duluth MN 55802        (800) 247-6789

◆ **Physical**: *Auto/Body Checkup* (W3.85, 15–20 min); *Fit to Be Interviewed* (W3.89, 45 min); *Consciousness-Raising Diet* (W3.87, 10–15 min).

◆ **Social**: *Health-Oriented People Hunt* (W3.75, 15—20 min), substituting attributes and questions that highlight interpersonal well-being issues; *Openness and Intimacy* (W3.91, 50–60 min).

◆ **Vocational**: *Compass* (W2.55, 30–60 min) helps put work into context; *Job Motivators* (W4.128, 40–45 min) explores the meaning of work.

◆ **Environmental**: Ardell's *Wellness Culture Test* (W3.80, 60–90 min) looks at the immediate environment and could be extended to a more global perspective.

◆ **Psychological**: *Polaroid Perspectives* (W3.94, 30–50 min) provides a developmental perspective; *Chemical Independence* (W3.86, 25–35 min) explores addictive patterns.

◆ **Spiritual**: *That's the Spirit!* (W3.92, 10–15 min).

◆ **Intellectual**: *50 Excuses for a Closed Mind* (W3.99, 5–15 min) could be expanded to include a presentation/discussion on nurturing a lively mind.

◆ **Emotional**: J*ournal to Music* (W3.90, 60–90 min) could be used for exploring emotional well-being; *The Feelings Factory* (W3.101, 2–3 min) is a related group energizer; *Self-Esteem Grid* (W4.123, 45–50 min) looks at another component of mental health.

Add appropriate group energizers as desired and finish with *Closing Statements* (W3.95, 10–30 min) or for a multisession course, *Health Report Card* (W3.98, 25–30 min).

## ▨ Healthy Eating Habits Mini-Workshop        (1.25–2.5 hours)

You will no doubt be asked at some point, and perhaps often, to provide a session or workshop targeting the "shame and blame" issues of wellness: physical fitness, chemical use (alcohol/tobacco/drugs), nutrition/eating habits/weight control.

Since our general bias is always to present wellness in the whole person context, we would encourage you to start with a general wellness assessment like *Health Lifelines* (W3.83, 75–90 minutes) or the *Personal Wellness Wheel* (W3.79, 15–20 minutes) that allows participants to consider these problematic areas in relationship to wider health and wholeness concerns, balanced with their self-care strengths and positive behaviors.

*Wellness 3* includes several nonjudgmental exercises you can group together as a mini-workshop on eating patterns for everyone—not only the overweight. Start with *My Mother Says* (W3.73a, 10–15 min), inviting participants to focus on food and eating-related messages they heard in their childhood and adolescence.

This personal exploration and sharing should level the playing field. Then break up into small groups and analyze the nutritional value and calorie count of a favorite meal using *Galloping Gourmet* (W3.78, 20–30 min). Follow this eye-opening experience with Dr Christopher's *Consciousness-Raising Diet* (W3.87, 10–15 minutes) and its five memorable questions.

Include some energy breaks like the empowering *Breathing Elements* (W3.100, 5 min) or the supportive *Waves* (W3.107, 5–10 min). *Noontime Energizers* (W1.33, 5–10 min), with its emphasis on identifying and satisfying all types of hungers, might be an enlightening addition if you have time.

The icebreaker *Sabotage and Self-Care* (W3.73b, 10–15 min) can be easily transformed into a thoughtful closing exercise that allows folks to acknowledge the difficulty of sustaining new patterns. Or use *Closing Statements* (W3.95, 10–30 min), which is generic enough to stimulate sharing of positive insights as well as planning for problem-oriented behavior change. If you'd rather end on a less serious note, try *Fortune Cookies* (W3.97, 15–20 min).

## WINNING COMBINATIONS                                              WELLNESS 4

### ▓ Health and Lifestyle Mini-Workshops                            (60–90 min)
You can use the film *Health and Lifestyle* (W4.117, 60–90 min) as a centerpiece for a mini-workshop on various wellness topics. The film provides an excellent overview of wellness concepts and provides a nice introduction for a special-emphasis presentation. Mix and match exercises from this and other volumes of the *Structured Exercises* series for thematic presentations on topics such as:

◆ Whole Person Wellness

◆ Wellness with a Stress Management/Relaxation Focus

◆ Habit Control: Nutrition, Smoking, Alcohol Use

◆ Cardiovascular Disease Prevention

See the outlines on p. 36–37 of *Wellness 4* for details. The chalktalk notes and process design of this exercise are excellent, with or without the film.

### ▓ Health Risks and Lifestyle Choices Presentation                (60–90 min)
Follow the process described in *Health and Lifestyle* (W4.117, 60–90 min) to explore the issues of stress, lifestyle, and risk factors. Use the icebreaker *Hearts at Risk* (W4.111, 10–15 min) for introductions and a warm-up to the topic of risk factors for cardiovascular disease, or try *Wellness Emblem* (W4.114, 15–20 min) for a more generic wellness orientation.

Don't miss the suggestion to stop the film and practice Herbert Benson's *Relaxation Response.* For a more extended closure/planning segment, add *Beat the Odds* (W4.130, 10–15 min) or *So What?* (S4.131, 10–15 min).

### ▓ Wellness Presentation Focus: Self-Esteem                       (1–2 hours)
Self-esteem is a key component of well-being, an essential ingredient for responsible self-care. Start with the icebreaker *Wellness Emblem* (W4.114, 15–20 min) or the self-care introduction *Decades* (W4.120, 15–20 min).

Once participants are tuned in to some of their personal wellness history, focus in on the issues of self-esteem using the checklists and process in *Self-Esteem Grid,* (W4.123, 45–50 min). If you want to extend the depth of your presentation by expanding on the issues of stress and self-esteem, use *The Fourth Source of Stress* (S2.42, 45–60 min).

Include some esteem-building energizers at appropriate points in the workshop. *Megaphone* (W1.32, 5–10 min), *Cheers!* (W2.64, 10–15 min), and *Get Off My Back!* (S1.29, 2 min) would fit well.

Close with the affirming process *Whisper Circle* (W4.134, 10–15 min). Don't forget to step in the circle yourself for some positive feedback.

---

### ▓ Play for the Health of It Workshop          (90 min–3 hours)

Use *Let's Play* (W4.127, 40–45 min) to put together a wellness training module for *Type As* and other over-responsible folks, like professional helpers, who are likely to turn wellness into work.

Supplement the exercise with as many playful, on-the-spot exercises as possible. There are some great ones in this volume: *12 Days of Wellness* (W4.135, 5 min), *Clapdance* (W4.138, 5–10 min), *Joke Around* (W4.140, 5 min), *New Sick Leave Policy* (W4.141, 5 min); as well as several in other *Structured Exercises* volumes: *Humorous Interludes* (S1.19, 5–10 min), *Month of Fundays*(S2.50, 20–30 min), *The Garden*(S2.63, 5 min), *Groans and Moans* (S3.103, 5–10 min), *Red Rover* (W1.34, 5–15 min), *Outrageous Episodes* (W3.104, 5–10 min).

If you have time for a longer workshop, add another creative content segment. *Whole Person Potpourri* (W4.116, 75–90 min) uses a playful approach to defining whole person well-being and developing innovative strategies to move toward that vision of health. Or launch the group on an playful exercise adventure with *Take A Walk!* (W4.121, 45–60 min).

Close with *Work of Art*(W4.133, 30 min), where participants create personal "pop art" sculptures symbolizing their enlightened understanding of wellness.

## WINNING COMBINATIONS                                       WELLNESS 5

### ▓ EAP and Health Promotion Presentations          (30–90 min)

If you are charged with promoting a wellness program or introducing EAP services in a workplace, a participatory learning experience is the most effective motivational tool available. Using the structured exercises in this volume you can spice up your marketing campaign as you get people actively involved in self-care issues. Consider using one of these approaches.

#### FITNESS FOCUS ▓

When it come to getting people geared up about fitness, it's tough to beat the *Healthy Exercise* (W5.158, 20–60 min) video/reflection/discussion process, which features ordinary folk—rather than fitness freaks—struggling to get/stay healthy.

The 60-minute process includes an icebreaker, personal reflection worksheets, small group sharing, and a planning process, as well as a brief visualization/ relaxation routine. If healthy eating is a potential hook to capture participants, try the unusual and affirming *Mealtime Meditation* (W5.157, 10–15 min).

#### MENTAL HEALTH FOCUS ▓

Motivating people to seek help with personal or family problems is no picnic, but it is possible. Begin the session with introductions, using the format from *I See Myself* (W5.145c, 5 min). Then engage people in defining mental health and recognizing common mental health problems using *Mental Health Index* (W5.161, 30–45 min). As part of *Step 6,* distribute information about EAP services or upcoming wellness programs.

Since relationship dynamics and work issues are such important components of mental well-being, try *Relationship Report Card* (W5.163, 30–40 min) and/or *Work APGAR* (W5.154, 10–15 min) if you have time.

---

Close with the intriguing floral essences metaphor *Self-Care Bouquet* (W5.169, 20–30 min).

If you have time for a group energizer, introduce the *Cleansing Breath* (W5.172, 3 min) or the *Personal Vitality Kit* (W5.177, 5–10 min) to stimulate creative self-care habits.

## ▧ Risk Factors and Self-Care Workshop			(90 min to 2 hrs)

If you're looking for a new approach to wellness, consider using the *Family Health Tree* (W5.150, 50–60 min) as the focal point for a workshop on personal health promotion. Most folks are intrigued by their family history, but very few have ever considered their heritage exclusively from a health perspective.

To set the tone for personal exploration of well-being, begin with *Health Transcript* (W5.147, 15–20 min), which challenges participants to assess all dimensions of their health—physical, mental, spiritual, relational, emotional, leisure. This whole person base will help people tune in to the wide variety of health issues that may emerge as they draw their family medical (and psycho-social) history.

◈ Since most families will reveal history of heart disease, you may want to include *Imagery for a Healthy Heart* (W5.159, 10–15 min) as a skill-building component of your presentation/workshop. Nearly everyone would benefit from a daily dose of this powerful, preventive, healing visualization.

Close the session with a reminder about the impact of our day to day behavior choices as they interact with our genetic and environmental heritage. Use the worksheet and open-ended format of *If . . . Then* (W5.167, 15–20 min) to help people project negative consequences of their health history and current health patterns. Then distribute a second *If . . . Then* worksheet and challenge people to imagine more positive health outcomes—and strategies they might use to reach them.

As a last hurrah, join in a group affirmation of the wellness lifestyle, using *Choose Wellness Anyway* (W5.171, 3–5 min).

If you're adventurous, lead the group in a rousing chorus of "If You're Healthy and You Know It" from *Healthy Singalong* (W5.174, 3–5 min) as an icebreaker, or after the *Health Transcripts*.

© 1995 Whole Person Press 210 W Michigan Duluth MN 55802		(800) 247-6789

# 4
# Editors' Choice

The editors of the *Structured Exercises in Stress Management* and *Wellness Promotion* series have chosen several exercises in each volume as favorites. After more than twenty years of teaching about stress and wellness, we know that these are truly gems—so we gave them our four-star rating. When you need something in a hurry that is guaranteed to work well with nearly any group, trust these four-star *Editors' Choices*.

Nancy Loving Tubesing, EdD
Donald A Tubesing, PhD
Sandy Stewart Christian, MSW

© 1995 Whole Person Press 210 W Michigan Duluth MN 55802          (800) 247-6789

| STRESS 2 | PAGE | EDITORS' CHOICE |
|---|---|---|
| **39 Four Quadrant Questions** | 9 | This two-part exercise draws on the resources of the group and is easy to adapt to your content. Always works well. (15–20 min, 10–15 min) |
| **42 The Fourth Source of Stress** | 17 | Self-esteem is a key source of stress—and a potential coping tool. Effective checklist and self-discovery process. (45–60 min) |
| **45 Back to the Drawing Board** | 32 | We use this right brain process periodically with our own staff to monitor stress levels and affirm coping efforts. It's a real winner! (50–75 min) |
| **47 Circuit Overload** | 46 | Easy, graphic, dependable warm-up for any stress presentation. (15–20 min) |
| **48 I've Got Rhythm** | 49 | This classic from the original *Stress Skills* workshop always produces new insights. (15–20 min) |
| **51 The Worry Stopper** | 64 | Everyone can identify with this universal stressor and quickly master the worry-stopper model. (30–40 min) |
| **53 Attitude Adjustment Hour** | 73 | One of our favorite techniques for demonstrating the role of perception in creating and relieving stress. Especially fun for a group that knows each other and can practice the technique together later. (25–35 min) |
| **57 The ABC's of Time** | 92 | Time management is always a hot topic for stress courses. This process is based on Alan Lakein's *How to Get Control of Your Time and Your Life.* (40–50 min) |
| **60 Goals, Obstacles and Actions** | 102 | A thorough planning process geared toward behavioral change. (60 min) |
| **63 The Garden** | 113 | This parable on play is our most frequently requested reading. (5 min) |

## STRESS 3 PAGE                     EDITORS' CHOICE

© 1995 Whole Person Press 210 W Michigan Duluth MN 55802        (800) 247-6789

| STRESS 4 | PAGE | EDITORS' CHOICE |
|---|---|---|

© 1995 Whole Person Press 210 W Michigan Duluth MN 55802          (800) 247-6789

| **WELLNESS 1** | PAGE | **EDITORS' CHOICE** |
|---|---|---|
| **2 Two-Minute Mill** | 5 | Like the two-minute drill in football, this is the time for lively action and risk-taking. The quick pace catches people off guard and gets the team moving quickly. Easy to adapt to the issues/location of any group. (10–15 min) |
| **6 Whole Person Health Appraisal** | 17 | Terrific whole-person health assessment in a memorable format. Participants identify personal health risk areas after taking their whole person (physical, mental, emotional, social, spiritual, lifestyle) "temperature." (20–30 min) |
| **10 Health/Illness Images** | 38 | Don considers this exercise his most powerful process for helping people uncover hidden meanings of health and illness and how these symbols shape lifestyle choices. (90 min) |
| **11 The Marathon Strategy** | 49 | Nearly everyone can identify with this familiar metaphor and apply it to their own self-care patterns. (15 min) |
| **17 Marco Polo** | 70 | This engaging film about curiosity always produces new insights and thought-provoking discussion about mental health as a component of wellness. (15–20 min) |
| **19 Interpersonal Needs** | 81 | Explore relationships as a source of well-being using an intriguing grid. Challenges participants to analyze their interpersonal needs and sources of support. (60–90 min) |
| **21 Spiritual Pilgrimage** | 94 | With a willing group this sharing of personal spiritual journeys is a very fruitful exploration of a key component of wellness. (20–30 min) |
| **25 Personal Prescription** | 110 | Quick, simple commitment to action technique. We use it all the time, with adaptations to match the topic or audience. (5–10 min) |
| **26 Meet the New Me** | 112 | A remnant of the original *WellAware* program, this closing ritual really packs a wallop. (10–15 min) |
| **30 Grabwell Grommet** | 121 | This clever portrayal of denial in action touches even the junk food junkies as it tickles the funny bone. (5 min) |
| **35 Singalong** | 132 | Music is a powerful vehicle for carrying profound messages. Nancy loves to get a group humming with these old favorites. (5 min) |
| **36 Slogans and Bumper Stickers** | 133 | A rousing success with any group that's willing to take a creative plunge. The resulting products often have practical value. (10–15 min) |

© 1995 Whole Person Press 210 W Michigan Duluth MN 55802          (800) 247-6789

| WELLNESS 3 | PAGE | EDITORS' CHOICE |
|---|---|---|

© 1995 Whole Person Press 210 W Michigan Duluth MN 55802        (800) 247-6789

# 5
# Especiallyfor
# the Workplace

Every volume in the *Stress* and *Wellness* series includes group processes that are especially effective in the workplace. If you would like to address issues unique to the job setting, or use techniques that work especially well with work teams, check out the exercises described in this index.

## STRESS 3       PAGE       ESPECIALLY FOR THE WORKPLACE

**74 Agenda Consensus**    4 Works well for staff meetings, too. (15 min)

**83 Job Descriptions**    40 Examines stress-provoking role stereotypes such as male-female, labor-management, supervisor-supervisee, etc. (60 min)

**88 Corporate Presentation**    66 Participants give themselves a lecture about the ten best methods for managing stress. (20–30 min)

**90 Conflict Management**   73 Applicable to any work setting. Be sure to customize for your audience. (60 min)

**94 Closing Formation**    97 Nice way to spread the insights around the group and provide positive closure. (10–30 min)

**97 My Stress Reduction Program**    107 Comprehensive planning process will appeal to straight line thinkers. Build a session around it. (20–30 min)

**107 You're Not Listening!** 129 Always a hit with work groups. (5–10 min)


## STRESS 4       PAGE       ESPECIALLY FOR THE WORKPLACE

**117 On the Job Stress Grid**    25 Identify job stress and coping options. Chalktalk and worksheet grid covering three sources of job stress: relationships, environment, expectations. (25–40 min)

**121 A Good Stress Manager**    49 Focus on coping attitudes/behaviors using the management metaphor and a group-generated assessment tool. (30–60 min)

**122 Obligation Overload**    55 Standing up to pressure; saying YES and NO! Use *Merry-Go-Round* (S4.139) as a lively warm-up/demonstration. (45 min)

**126 Go for the Gold**    73 Personal goal-setting techniques. (30–40 min)

**133 Pat on the Back**    107 Affirmation experience for work groups. (20–30 min)

**137 How to Swim with Sharks**    118 Managers love this reading. (5 min)


## STRESS 5       PAGE       ESPECIALLY FOR THE WORKPLACE

**146 Badge of My Profession**    4 Suitable for any work group interested in getting better acquainted. (15–20 min)

---

© 1995 Whole Person Press 210 W Michigan Duluth MN 55802      (800) 247-6789

**149 Pace Setters**          12  Great way to get acquainted and pave the way for
                                  a session on stress. (5–10 min)

**151 The Hardiness Factor**  17  Powerful assessment tool, likely to promote rich
                                  discussion about ways to become more stress-
                                  resistant. (30–40 min)

**152 Lifetrap 5:**           22  Relevant and useful for working women in any
**Superwoman Stress**             occupation. (60–90 min)

**156 Managing**              49  Perfect for a brown-bag lunch seminar. Adaptable
**Job Stress**                    for shorter or longer sessions. (20–60 min)

**159 Stress Management**     59  Rich variety of techniques packed into a short time.
**Alphabet**                      Practical and fun. (50–60 min)

**162 Eating under Stress**   76  Job stress can alter eating patterns, so consider
                                  including this exercise in your worksite wellness
                                  program. (40–45 min)

**164 Remote Control**        91  Natural skills can promote self-control at work as
                                  well as at home. (5–10 min)

**169 Key Learning**         108  A door-opening process for closure and planning in
                                  any training event. (20–30 min)

**171 Anti-Stress**          113  A healthy break for an extended meeting or training
**Coffee Break**                  event. (10–15 min)

**176 Stress Squeezers**     124  This tried and true technique for relieving stress
                                  and tension is perfect for the workplace.
                                  (10–15 min)

**177 Superman**             126  Humorous approach reduces tension about work
                                  performance and perfectionism. (5–10 min)

**180 Try, Try Again**       133  Everyone can identify with the fly in this parable.
                                  (5 min)

© 1995 Whole Person Press 210 W Michigan Duluth MN 55802        (800) 247-6789

© 1995 Whole Person Press 210 W Michigan Duluth MN 55802      (800) 247-6789

| WELLNESS 4 | PAGE | ESPECIALLY FOR THE WORKPLACE |
|---|---|---|
| **109c TP Tales** | 4 | Offbeat icebreaker that loosens up a group. Works especially well in medical settings. (2 min per person) |
| **111 Hearts at Risk** | 6 | This inviting process introduces the issue of risk factors and general health concerns related to heart disease. (10–15 min) |
| **117 Health and Lifestyle** | 33 | Although this film is somewhat dated, it is still valuable for its wide view of wellness issues. The *Variations* section has lots of suggestions for special emphasis programs you can tailor to fit your setting and the specific wellness issues of your training (eg, alcohol use, cardiovascular risks, stress management, self-care). (60–90 min) |
| **121 Take a Walk!** | 52 | Great kickoff for a workplace walking campaign. Models support and creativity as components of a successful exercise program. (45–60 min) |
| **128 Job Motivators** | 85 | Use the *Wheel of Fortune* (W4.113) as a warm-up to this in-depth examination of needs and motivations. Participants determine their personal priorities for job satisfaction and compare them to their current job setting. (40–45 min) |
| **131 Discoveries** | 100 | Through the use of an in-session insight journal, this process models a potent self-care tool—periodic reflection and goal-setting. Works best in a longer workshop or multi-session course. (20–30 min) |
| **141 New Sick Leave Policy** | 125 | This employee benefit spoof should bring down the house. (5 min) |
| **144 Twenty Reasons** | 132 | To close your session, try a variation of this exercise where the group brainstorms twenty reasons why other employees should take your course. Bask in the responses and then use them in your next marketing campaign. (5 min) |

## WELLNESS 5      PAGE      ESPECIALLY FOR THE WORKPLACE

© 1995 Whole Person Press 210 W Michigan Duluth MN 55802     (800) 247-6789

# 6
# Tips
# for Trainers

The essays included in this section originally appeared as *Tips for Trainers* in the ten volumes of the *Structured Exercises in Stress* and *Wellness* series. No matter whether you are a novice health educator or a senior consultant, you'll find practical ideas that will enhance your effectiveness in preparation and presentation.

## CREATING THE RHYTHM OF A
## PRESENTATION OR WORKSHOP
STRESS 1

Most of the longer (40–90 min) exercises in the *Structured Exercises* volumes use a time-tested pattern for guaranteeing participant involvement. The magic is in the rhythm—which you can use in designing your own presentations and workshops.

◆ **Warm-up.** Start with some kind of process that invites participants to get acquainted with the topic—and with each other. When you're planning a one-hour session, this icebreaker needs to be short and sweet. For a longer workshop you can afford to spend 15–45 minutes in a warm-up activity.

In either case, the *content* and *process* of the warm-up should lead naturally into the next learning segment. Don't use a generic icebreaker! Make each moment an integral part of the themes you hope to cover.

◆ **Content Presentation.** If you are planning just one session with a group, choose a single focus for your major content presentation. You may want to provide a comprehensive picture of the sources of stress and resources for coping. Or you may choose to focus on stress assessment only, or general coping strategies, or a single skill as an antidote to stress.

Usually you still want to tailor your content in response to the expressed concerns of the group, but introducing a new perspective of stress and/or challenging the audience through consciousness-raising are also effective approaches.

◆ **Sharing.** Trainers typically judge this the riskiest component of the learning experience. We trainers somehow feel that if we are not talking all the time, demonstrating our expertise, we are not doing an adequate job. In fact, for many participants, the chance to compare notes with others is often the most fruitful part of the session.

At minimum, allow for several brief exchanges where people share insights with a neighbor. Better yet, build into every 60 minutes of presentation at least 15 minutes of small group conversation, with every person guaranteed at least 4–5 minutes of "air" time.

In some settings—for example, an intact staff with power differentials, or mixed client/staff groups—you may need to provide more structure about appropriate disclosure, but for most groups, participants naturally tend to share at their own level of comfort and propriety.

◆ **Planning/Commitment.** This is the bottom line in training. Make sure everyone leaves the session with at least one clear idea about how they can implement what they have learned—and with the resolve to do so.

For half-day or longer workshops, use this same general pattern at a more leisurely pace. Each 60–90 minute segment needs a rhythm similar to that outlined above. And the entire workshop should flow with a wider rhythm progressing from warm-up to closure, with several periods of reflection and planning.

You will also need to include more energizers and activities to change the pace at strategic points. Be sure to provide some measure of closure before breaks and warm-ups after breaks.

In the longer workshop or several-session course you can afford to be more change-oriented and spend longer time periods for skill-building, goal-setting, and planning.

© 1995 Whole Person Press 210 W Michigan Duluth MN 55802      (800) 247-6789

## HOW TO GET PEOPLE INVOLVED                          STRESS 2

As you will notice in just a cursory glance through these handbooks, we believe strongly in designing educational experiences that actively involve participants in the learning process. When you draw on the resources of the group in your presentations, you empower people.

For most trainers, giving up the "authority" implicit in the typical lecture format is a risky proposition. We're afraid that we won't be perceived as an "expert," so we lecture, entertain, and keep the focus on ourselves. Yet, if your goal is truly to help people change, information is not enough. Praise from your audience is not enough. What really counts are the discoveries participants make about their own unhealthy patterns and the choices they make to manage their stress more effectively.

Certainly you have expertise to offer your audiences. But the greatest gift you can give is to tap into the wisdom and creativity of individuals and the group as a whole. Their knowledge base, experiences, and insights will enrich and expand your expertise. Asking for significant input can also help you tune in to the specific needs of your participants and tailor your comments, examples, and activities to meet them more precisely.

Your task is to appeal to people with different learning styles, using a wide variety of strategies to get them involved. In whole person learning, the questions are as important as the content. Don't be intimidated by the small number of stubborn rationalists who may sit with their arms crossed, waiting for the "right" answers in outline form. In stress management there are no right answers, no simple solutions, and no single path.

Several "projective" exercises where major content is provided by large or small group discussion are included in *Stress 2*. We hope you will stretch yourself and experiment with some of these:

> *Four Quadrant Questions* (S2.39)
> *Exclusive Interview* (S2.41)
> *Consultants Unlimited* (S2.52)
> *Personal/Professional Review* (S2.58)
> *Manager of the Year* (S2.59)
> *25 Words or Less* (S2.61)
> *Stress and Coping Journal* (S2.62)

Individual reflection processes provide another vehicle for provoking insights and for stimulating participation. The following exercises in *Stress 2* use "empty" worksheets that call on the individual's resources to generate examples, assessments, strategies, etc.

> *Back to the Drawing Board* (S2.45)
> *Circuit Overload* (S2.47)
> *Month of Fundays* (S2.50)
> *The Worry Stopper* (S2.51)

Don't worry. If lecturing is your thing, and content is your focus, you'll find plenty of chalktalk notes and content outlines in most exercises. But please do accept our invitation to experiment with participant empowerment by trusting your audience—get them involved!

---

## FRESH APPROACHES TO STRESS                                          STRESS 3

The vast majority of stress management presentations begin with some comprehensive, generic introduction to stress from either the physical or the emotional perspective. Moving from the general to the specific is often an effective way to engage participants, so we have included several exercises in *Stress 3* that offer the broad view:

> *Spice or Arsenic?* (S3.79)
> *Drainers and Energizers* (S3.80)
> *Lifetrap 3: Sick of Change* (S3.82)
> *S.O.S for Stress* (S3.86)
> *Corporate Presentation* (S3.88)

If, on the other hand, you're interested in trying a really novel approach in your next presentation, why not choose a more specific starting point to "hook" your audience, and then generalize about stress and coping from the data generated by the group? Start by vividly illustrating the stress reaction using one of these effective demonstrations:

> *Under Fire* (S3.73b)
> *Marauders* (S3.75)

Then try one or more of the following exercises as a centerpiece for your workshop. Draw your generalizations from data generated by the group, weaving the participants' insights into your chalktalks and introductions to activities.

◆ **STRESS focus**. Explore one of three specific sources of stress common to most people: manipulation, role stereotyping, or rejection.

> *On the Spot* (S3.80)
> *Job Descriptions* (S3.83)
> *The Last Christmas Tree* (S3.84)

◆ **COPING focus**. Generate specific stress clusters and plan coping strategies. Or introduce one of two key skills with applications at work and home: conflict management or active listening.

> *Stress Clusters Clinic* (S3.87)
> *Conflict Management* (S3.90)
> *Stop Look and Listen* (S3.92)

◆ **RELAXATION focus**. Experiment with one of the three basic forms of relaxation: meditation/guided imagery, autogenic sequences, or massage.

> *Centering Meditation* (S3.93)
> *Warm Hands* (S3.105)
> *Pushing My Buttons* (S3.108)

Variety is the spice of life (see S3.79)! We hope this volume will inspire you to turn on your own creativity and experiment with some fresh approaches to teaching about stress.

© 1995 Whole Person Press 210 W Michigan Duluth MN 55802        (800) 247-6789

## WHAT? SO WHAT? NOW WHAT?                                    STRESS 4

*So What?* (S4.131) could be used as a model for planning any presentation or workshop.

◈ **WHAT** do you want people to learn? WHAT do they need/want? WHAT special focus will be important as you tailor your presentation to the group? WHAT information is essential? WHAT resources are available to you and to your participants?

◈ **SO WHAT?** This is the relevance question. How can you make the concepts come alive for participants and help people apply this information to their own situation? Start with yourself. What does this idea mean to you? How have you struggled with this issue? What strategies have you used in similar situations? What does the research say? Develop many personal examples for the content and concepts you are presenting.

◈ **NOW WHAT?** Information and reflection are key steps in the learning process, but the bottom line is action. As you plan, be sure to incorporate processes that will engage people in making plans for change. Include periodic exercises that ask questions like: What are the next steps that I need to take? What do I still need to learn?

Why not make a copy of the *So What?* worksheet on page 104 of *Stress 4* and use it when planning your next presentation?

*Stress 4* contains only a few full-session outlines (45–90 minutes). However, several of the short exercises (5–40 minutes) combine well for longer presentations and workshops.

Build a workshop around *Lifetrap 4: Good Grief* (S4.120) as described in the outline on p. 68. Or use *On the Job Stress Grid* (S4.117) as the centerpiece of a work stress presentation.

## TEN COMMANDMENTS FOR ETHICAL TRAINING          STRESS 5

Whatever your professional background, from business to psychology to nursing, as a trainer you have developed an internalized set of ethical principles that guide your work. These may be so basic to you that you take them for granted, but these guidelines are vital ingredients that undergird every presentation or workshop. The *Ten Commandments for Ethical Training* may provide a consciousness-raising reminder for you.

### Thou shalt do what thou said thou would do.

◈ It's tempting to offer the moon in order to close a juicy deal or to please a committee. Don't promise something you can't deliver.

◈ Show up early, know what you're doing, and do what you promised. Always have a backup plan. If an emergency makes it impossible for you to be there, provide a qualified substitute.

◈ Be clear about the training agenda—and stick to it.

### Thou shalt use the power of the podium with care.

◈ Be cognizant of your influential position. Do not exploit the dependency and trust of participants. Respect their personal boundaries and need for privacy.

◈ Group dynamics can be dangerous. Encouragement and good-natured cajoling can help reluctant folks get over their anxiety, but never embarrass, manipulate, or coerce people into doing what doesn't feel good to them. For example, *Stress Management Alphabet* (S5.159) includes a group backrub that should be gracefully optional.

◈ Don't toot your own horn. Affirm the contributions of participants rather than your expertise. Emphasize the learning process rather than your teaching skills. It's okay to mention your products or services briefly, but don't push them.

### Thou shalt keep the group process safe for all.

◈ When planning a session, select activities that are suited to the setting and audience. Be cautious about using exercises in the workplace that may have repercussions on the individuals involved. Intense personal reflection or deep sharing probably don't belong in the workplace, except in voluntary self-help groups with trained leadership.

◈ Create a respectful, safe environment where people are accepted and not put down. Make sure the process is inclusive of all people—and that their rights are protected.

### Honor all thy participants.

◈ Show respect for diverse racial, ethnic, age, status, and gender groups. Use inclusive language. Keep your examples respectful and inclusive. Maintain strict confidentiality.

◈ Be careful with humor. NEVER tell an off-color joke or use coarse language. Sexual innuendo is always offensive to someone. Please refrain. Make yourself, not participants, the target of any contextual humor.

◈ Don't let one or two people dominate the group or cause you to stray from your agenda.

◆ Listen with care to comments and questions from the audience. Always restate the contribution so everyone knows what was said—and the individual feels heard.

**Thou shalt not allow bloodletting.**

◆ Set limits for appropriate self-disclosure.

◆ Avoid confrontation or opening old wounds (personal or organizational) unless this is explicitly part of your contract.

◆ Finish what you start, support participants throughout the process, and provide closure.

**Thou shalt refrain from involvements with participants.**

◆ Maintain professional boundaries. Be friendly and personable, but limit socializing with participants before, during, and after training. Romantic or sexual intimacy with participants is a violation of their boundaries, no matter how willing they may be.

**Thou shalt not steal the work of thy colleagues.**

◆ Give credit where credit is due. Don't take another trainer's paradigm and present it as your own. An idea may not care who its owner is, but people who have invested their professional lives in developing ground-breaking concepts, clear paradigms, clever turns of phrase, field-tested assessments, concise checklists, touching stories, provocative questions, or elegant graphic representations of complex issues deserve to be acknowledged as the originators.

◆ Be sure that every handout you distribute includes a proper citation of the source and identification of whose creative work it represents.

**Thou shalt represent thyself authentically.**

◆ Make up your own stories, jokes, examples, and approaches rather than "borrowing" the best of others. Develop a distinctive style of presentation that represents your own creative uniqueness.

◆ Correct any misleading or inaccurate description of your background or credentials.

**Thou shalt set reasonable fees for your products and services.**

◆ Give people what they are paying for—a service tailored to their specific needs and interests—rather than a canned program, or a clone of what you have developed for another group.

◆ Make your training affordable for a wide range of groups. Non-profits and small businesses need training just as badly as the Fortune 500.

**Thou shalt ask permission to borrow intellectual property.**

◆ Know and respect copyright laws and conventions. It is illegal to photocopy and distribute charts, checklists, concept summaries, articles, tips, cartoons, or any other material in print without specific permission from the publisher of the original work. Such permission is usually easy to obtain from the Permissions Department of the magazine, journal, or book publisher. In your written request, include information about how you plan to use the material (in a handout, publishing it in a workbook, adapting it for a worksheet, etc) and the number of reproductions you plan to make. Some publishers have different guidelines for profit and non-profit uses. Allow 30 days for a response. Always be sure to use the proper reprint citation on every reproduction.

◆ Remember, duplicating audio or video cassettes is also illegal and un-ethical— no matter how easy it is! Most videotapes are intended for individual viewing only. Check with the publisher/producer for information on licensing agreements for classroom/workshop use or wide broadcast on closed-circuit or cable TV. The Whole Person video series used in *Managing Job Stress* (S5.156) for example, is sold with rights for classroom (but not broadcast) use included in the price.

**Thou shalt remember these commandments and keep them holy.**

Give yourself a periodic ethical check-up by reviewing the *Ten Commandments* every six months. Share them with your colleagues and let these guidelines serve as a stimulus for thoughtful discussion about the complex ethical issues involved in training.

## HOW TO DESIGN A WELLNESS
## PRESENTATION, WORKSHOP, OR COURSE                     WELLNESS 1

No matter what your background, putting together a wellness presentation can be a real challenge. The concept is vague and crosses boundaries of several professions. Goals and objectives are tough to pin down and measure. Wellness events attract a wide cross-section of people with dissimilar and sometimes conflicting agendas. But the rewards of turning people on to healthier lifestyles can be most gratifying.

Where should you start?

Successful training starts with the *first contact,* when you begin the creative process of clarifying the client's needs, reviewing your expertise and resources to determine how they might match this agenda, and planning tentative content and process pieces to accomplish the goals.

◈ From the first conversation, start *clarifying expectations.* Does your client really want a fitness program? A stress management workshop? A course in health risks? A program for eliminating negative health behaviors (eg, drug use, smoking, etc)? A morale-booster or team-building experience?

◈ Get to know as much as you can about your *potential audience.* Is the group likely to include wellness old-timers looking for affirmation and story-swapping? Or neophytes looking for opportunities to learn and grow? Or resident cynics? Or a target population who will feel blamed and shamed? Or others who will be looking for concrete answers to very painful issues/problems? Will the group be homo-geneous or cross supervision or department lines? Now is the time to speak up if you have recommendations about who should be included.

◈ Make sure you *represent yourself well* in this initial conversation. You may be eager to please the prospective client—and eager for the paycheck—but don't promise more than you can deliver. Be clear about what you have to offer. Where possible, help translate the stated agenda into concepts and processes that fit you expertise. Steer the conversation towards areas that match your passions and experience. But don't push this too far, or you're headed for disappointment. If the topic or the group or the style the client is proposing doesn't fit you, bow out gracefully—and suggest someone else who might fit the bill.

Be sure to *keep good notes* of this initial (and all other) conversations. Jot down the specific issues, goals, and objectives discussed, using the client's language and metaphors. Note any process/content ideas you have as the discussion progresses. Keep track of names and any other relevant data (date, location, fees, etc). You may want to want to develop a standard "initial contact" sheet for recording this information, and to jog your memory about items that should be discussed. Start a file folder right away so you'll have some place to put these notes for later reference and to collect ideas that might fit this presentation.

The next step in planning is to develop a tentative outline for the training. This is the time for exploration and creativity.

◈ Start with a *self-inventory.* Review your notes from previous training events, looking for a skeleton outline you can adapt to this situation. Which of your polished training modules will mesh with the client's agenda? What would you most like to teach about? What ideas and issues are turning your crank these days? Go with your strengths—those are the qualities that make you an effective trainer. But every new request is also a creative opportunity for you to learn and grow.

◈ This is also the time for research. Check in with the experts in print or person to update your information base. Brainstorm creative strategies for tackling the issues. Browse through *Structured Exercises* volumes looking for intriguing approaches with goals and objectives that match your client's. Watch for clever titles and processes that complement your style. Scout for related news stories, anecdotes, cartoons, illustrations. Collect them all. When your agenda is filled to overflowing with powerful processes—and your file folder for the event is plump with ideas—put it away for a few days. Let it incubate.

Separate the creative/expansive part of your planning from the evaluative.

◈ After a day or two, go back and review your design—*then cut it in half!* In our efforts to please clients and to keep anxiety in abeyance, most trainers try to crowd too much into their presentations. Don't do it! Pare your outline down now— then plan to keep some of the "out-take" modules in the wings for reinsertion into your presentation if something goes more quickly than you expected. Now you'll have a design that lets you know clearly where you're heading, but will be flexible enough to adapt on the spot.

◈ Circle back and *check your final product.* Does your design meet your client's goals? Will the content and process address the varying agendas of your audience? Does your plan fit you and satisfy your expectations? If so, you're well on the way to a successful training.

All that's left is practicing with your new material, trying on the concepts and processes, generating personal examples and continuing to collect the illustrations that will help you stay fresh. By the time you get to the podium, the hardest part of the work is done! Good luck.

© 1995 Whole Person Press 210 W Michigan Duluth MN 55802        (800) 247-6789

## USING A WHOLE PERSON MODEL
## IN PREPARATION AND IMPLEMENTATION                    WELLNESS 2

When we first joined the fledgling wellness movement back in the early 1970s we found ourselves prophets crying out in the wilderness of the medical establishment, challenging physicians and health educators and patients to return to a more wholistic view of health. The concept of whole person well-being—body, mind, and spirit integrated in a desire for health and wholeness—is as old as history, from the ancient orient to Alexandria and Athens to the native Americas.

Today nearly everyone is on board with the concept of health as a whole person issue, and you will want to consider this as you plan and present your training events. Our whole person logo can serve as a reminder to attend to the *physical* (dancing person), *mental* (lightbulb), *emotional* (heart), *interpersonal* (dancing folk), and *spiritual* (candle) dimensions of wellness, as well as to the *lifestyle* choices that connect and draw together all these dimensions into a unified whole (outlines of the circle and its component parts).

This logo can also remind you to attend to the whole person as you prepare your learning experiences. No matter how homogeneous a group seems, don't be fooled. Participants come to your presentations with widely different needs, life experiences, attitudes, knowledge bases, and expectations. Preparation is somewhat easier if you can get a sense of this variety beforehand, and plan your processes and illustrations to match the group in general, but you also need to prepare for the individuals in particular. Two strategies are of particular importance.

First, tune up your projective and empathic skills. As you prepare each segment of your presentation, mentally insert yourself into the life situations of several potential participants. Then think through your design and imagine how that person might respond to the issues you will be raising or the activities you are planning. How will each one respond to the reflection and analysis you will be guiding? What kinds of concerns will they be sharing with others in pairs or small groups? This mental warm-up should help you identify with your audience—and help you choose appropriate examples and illustrations.

Second, anticipate that your group will include a variety of folks with dramatically different learning styles. Many will be able to absorb and process information primarily through their auditory channel, so your lectures and group discussion may be effective with them. Other participants will take in and process information primarily visually. A-V resources and handouts will be more important to them. Still others learn primarily experientially. They will need movement, activity, simulations, demonstrations, practice for maximum learning. Your challenge is to vary your presentation style and processes enough to meet the needs of all.

If you use an introspective and analytical-type icebreaker like *Roundup* (W2.37a, 5–15 min), try closing with a more active and interpersonal closing experience like *Vital Signs* (W2.62, 10–15 min) or a creative planning exercise like *One-a-Day Plan* (W2.61, 10–30 min) or an unusual concept review like *Cheers!* (W2.64, 10–15 min). Make sure you include plenty of activities that illustrate or demonstrate your message.

Keep the logo in mind as you plan content and process that will:

◈ Energize the group through *physical* activity and demonstrations (dancing person).

---

◆ Challenge the intellect and tap into the creative potential of the *mental* dimension (lightbulb).

◆ Engage people's feelings on the *emotional* level (heart).

◆ Connect participants with each other through sharing and activities that affirm *interpersonal* needs and authenticate their individual experiences and varied perspectives (dancing folk).

◆ Reach the inner *spiritual* core that provides meaning, purpose, and the power to make healthy changes (candle).

◆ Assist participants in reviewing the past and envisioning positive futures in the integrative process of developing a healthier *lifestyle* (connecting and encircling lines).

The exercises in these volumes are designed with this whole person perspective of content and process, and give you some creative, field-tested tools to start with. When you bring your own whole person vision and special gifts to the preparation and training experience as well, your audiences will benefit from a dynamite formula for wellness training.

© 1995 Whole Person Press 210 W Michigan Duluth MN 55802        (800) 247-6789

## DEVELOPING MULTI-SESSION
## COURSES OR WORKSHOPS                                          WELLNESS 3

One-shot wellness presentations can be fun and motivating, but if you are interested in helping people make significant behavior change, you will need to plan an extended learning experience with skill practice during and between sessions, opportunities for mid-course evaluation and corrections, and lots of personal and interpersonal support. There are several effective models for longer learning experiences.

◆ **Course with 4–8 Sessions**. (6–16 hours)

This typical adult education model often features weekly meetings of 90 minutes to 2 hours and offers maximum responsiveness to participant needs as the trainer adjusts the course content and process from week to week to meet the expressed concerns of the group. Participants have an opportunity to implement and practice new behaviors between sessions and report back regularly on progress.

◆ **One- or Two-Day Workshop**. (8–16 hours)

The workshop setting allows larger blocks of time to develop key concepts, explore options, and make connections. This model tends to build group camaraderie quickly, without wasting time getting reacquainted and warmed up before each session. Unfortunately, there is no between-session opportunity for reflection and experimentation.

◆ **Combination Workshop/Course**. (9–20 hours)

Start with a half-day or full-day exploratory and goal-setting workshop (4–8 hours) with a 3–6 session follow-up. This model creates enough shared experience initially to solidify the group, yet still allows you to incorporate participant's individual goals in planning the remaining sessions.

Any of these models can work well. Choose the one that fits your setting, audience, and personal style. We have designed the *Structured Exercises* volumes to give you the resources you need, no matter what model you choose. The *Whole Person Wellness Presentation Plus* outline on p. 73 makes a good starting point for designing a multi-session course. Use the *Personal Wellness Wheel* (W3.79) or *Health Lifelines* (W3.83) for the first session. Compile suggestions from participants on their personal goals, then choose themes for the remaining sessions that address these issues. You may want to supplement the exercises in *Wellness 3* with thematic processes from other *Structured Exercises* volumes.

No matter what the model, in designing a wellness course or longer workshop, you need to incorporate all the content objectives in a sequence that takes advantage of the extended time period and flows naturally over the sessions, using processes that activate and reinforce healthy group dynamics. At the same time, you need to create each individual session with its own objectives and rhythms that maximize participant involvement.

◆ Begin with a welcoming icebreaker that helps people get acquainted and introduces some aspect of the course content. The *Icebreakers* section of every *Structured Exercises* volume has several topical warm-ups.

◆ Present the major content segment of the session. In the early part of the course, this may come from the *Wellness Exploration* section of *Structured Exercises.*

As the course progresses, you will want to focus on practical applications like those presented in the *Self-Care Strategies* section. Every volume of *Structured Exercises* includes in this section processes addressing physical (fitness, nutrition, relaxation), mental, emotional, spiritual, lifestyle, and self-care issues. Choose several that fit the goals of your group and plan sessions around them, using related icebreakers, planning processes, and group energizers.

◈ Schedule in time for personal reflection and application of the concepts you've presented. Nearly every *Structured Exercise* gives you a worksheet or handout to help people focus. Then be sure to allow time for sharing in small groups. This is really the heart of the learning process, the place where people test out their insights, clarify their goals, and learn from others.

◈ Every session should end with a concrete planning or application process where participants identify goals and next steps. Many of the designs in *Structured Exercises* have built-in closure processes, but you might want to check out the variety of options in the *Planning/Closure* sections.

◈ In a multi-session course, or between workshop days, be sure to assign some homework. This could take the form of skill practice, journaling, or tracking behaviors as outlined in *Daily Wellness Graph* (W3.96). Remember that it's what happens at home that will be the real measure of your success.

◈ Do take time at the end of every segment to summarize and provide transition. Polling the group for insights is a great way to do this. It gives people a chance to reinforce their learning, adds to the corporate wisdom, and gives you a final opportunity to fill in the gaps.

◈ Don't forget to check out the *Group Energizers* section for demonstrations and activities that can vividly illustrate key concepts and provide a change of pace.

◈ If relaxation/meditation skills are important to your agenda, teach a different type at every session and encourage participants to practice in between.

Or teach one key technique and practice it at every session.

At the final session of your course/workshop, take time to celebrate what you have shared together. *Health Report Card* (W3.98) allows participants an opportunity to give positive feedback on progress. *Fortune Cookies* (W3.97) is a more whimsical affirmation of best wishes for wellness.

As you plan, it's helpful to think in time modules, and then use these modules as mix and match building blocks. We tend to conceptualize in 45 minute blocks and many of the processes in the *Structured Exercises* volumes use this time frame. It's just about the time you'll need to introduce a concept, ask participants to reflect and apply it to their own life, and facilitate small group sharing to compare notes and receive support—with a few moments to elicit summary comments and insights. Toss in a group energizer or two, and you have an hour block. Icebreakers and planning processes usually take about 20 minutes, or half a module. Some of the extended reflection exercises and creative explorations take up to 90 minutes, or two modules. Start with a key exercise or two for each session, then supplement with other processes until you fill time blocks.

## A Note on Group Dynamics

At the beginning of each session, participants will need time to regroup, touch base, focus. During the first few sessions, use a structured approach to this warm-up time with a thematic icebreaker such as *My Mother Says* (W3.73a), *Part of Me* (W3.76), *Getting to Know You* (W3.77), *Galloping Gourmet* (W3.78), *Well Cards* (W3.82), or *Sabotage and Self-Care* (W3.73b).

In later sessions simple check-in "rounds" (eg, homework report, progress on goals) will work well. For efficiency and bonding you may want to use a buddy system where participants pair and share at the beginning of each meeting. Switch the pairings a couple of times during the course.

As people get to know each other better, you will need to allocate more time during the sessions for interaction. People will be eager to tell their success stories and to hear how others are doing. As respect for each other grows, participants will also ask for advice or encouragement.

## USING A-V MATERIAL EFFECTIVELY WELLNESS 4

All of the exercises in this and other volumes of the *Structured Exercises* series are based on the model of experiential learning—creating opportunities for participants to interact with the concepts and each other in meaningful ways. The lecture method is replaced with succinct chalktalks and facilitative questions that guide people to discover their own answers. The "authority" of the trainer is transformed into the "authority" of the individual's inner wisdom.

Within this overarching educational framework, there is plenty of latitude for using all types of resources from guest experts to overheads to hypercard stacks and interactive video. Different media formats can be extremely valuable adjuncts to your training, as long as you don't let technology interfere with the goal of experiential learning. As a trainer, you are not presenting a paper at a conference. You are engaging an audience in an educational process. There is nothing more deadly than the "professional" presentation featuring one text-filled blue slide after another. When you turn out the lights, the audience often tunes out—unless you have prepared them to stay involved.

*Health and Lifestyle* (W4.117, 60–90 min) is a good model for using audio-visual resources wisely, incorporating a short film as an information source and spring-board for structured personal reflection and group interaction.

Audio-visual materials can be potent tools when they are well-integrated into your training strategy. Here are a few tips for using media effectively in a training setting.

- ◆ **Match media to specific educational goals**. Import the experts or bring the real world into the training setting with video. Use it to introduce, reinforce, or sum-marize your content presentation, or to demonstrate a skill such as relaxation, stretching, or assertiveness.

- ◆ **Use A-V for variety**. As you try to appeal to the diverse learning styles of your audience, audio and visual resources effectively reach folks who learn best in those channels and provide a change of pace for everyone. A-V is a great way to inject some humor into your presentation, with cartoons on overheads or a Bill Cosby clip that illustrates a key point.

- ◆ **Technology can enhance your image**. In some settings you will want to incorporate A-V materials in your training just to raise your credibility. The medical establishment expects slides, so give them a few. But use them in a way that stimulates active involvement rather than passive participation. Corporate America may expect action-packed video or slick overheads. Nothing wrong with that—as long as you also invite your audience to connect what they see and hear with their own life situations. When a topic is controversial or difficult, it's sometimes wise to raise the issue through media. If there is resistance from the audience, you can play the "good guy" and let the "outside expert" take the flack.

Whenever you use A-V resources, be sure to fit the medium to your message and integrate it completely into your process design.

- ◆ If a video is supposed to deliver key content for the session, give people some warm-up that will engage their curiosity. Give them a list of things to watch for or intriguing questions that may be answered in the film. Brainstorm with the group beforehand what they imagine might be included in a film on this topic.

© 1995 Whole Person Press 210 W Michigan Duluth MN 55802 (800) 247-6789

◆ Stop a film in the middle and ask people to predict what will happen next. Or stop several times for written reflection (individuals) or discussion (pairs/small groups) of what participants have learned or how they identify with the issues raised. Or stop as appropriate during the film to practice a skill, apply a principle, discuss alternatives.

◆ At the end, review the content by soliciting comments from participants or presenting your own summary points.

◆ But don't stop there. Develop a worksheet and process tailored to the film and your audience. Help people apply what they have seen and heard to their own life situation. Use the *Health and Lifestyle* (W4.117) worksheet as a model.

A savvy trainer will also exercise some caution in using A-V resources. Forewarned is forearmed.

◆ Always preview media. Know what you're going to show. Check films for in(ex)-clusive language, stereotypes, diversity, appropriateness to the setting/audience.

◆ Expect something will go wrong. Be prepared. Don't depend on media services at the site to have everything in order. Go early and check out the equipment. If you are supplying your own equipment, make sure you have extra bulbs, long extension cords, etc.

◆ Always have a backup plan in case your A-V malfunctions.

A-V resources from posters to relaxation music to video to computer graphics can be powerful tools for learning. But don't be a slave to media. Remember—you and your participants are the best source of wisdom.

## USING YOUR SEVEN IQS                                          WELLNESS 5

Wellness is a complicated issue for most of us—evaluating lifestyle habits and getting motivated to change our patterns takes our best problem-solving skills. That's why *Seven Ways of Knowing* (W5.162) may be the most important process in *Wellness 5* for you as a trainer. Gardner's revolutionary concept of multiple intelligences challenges us as educators to examine our teaching style to make sure we are activating all types of intelligence in our program planning and presentation.

Start by looking closely at the seven types of intelligence described on pages 78–80 of *Wellness 5*. You probably engage several of these modes in any presentation— telling stories or jokes *(verbal/linguistic)*, inserting a puzzle or brain teaser for effect *(logical/mathematical)*, providing visual aids with charts, diagrams, slides, etc *(visual/spatial)*, and encouraging individual reflection and application of your content presentation *(intrapersonal)*. Most trainers these days provide at least a bit of time for small group discussion or sharing with a neighbor *(interpersonal)*, but rarely do trainers feel comfortable asking audiences to role play *(kinesthetic)*, or join in a *musical/rhythmic* exercise.

Unfortunately, most adults rarely exercise these last two modes—having been socialized to leave these areas to the professionals. Perhaps your most potent tools as a trainer are the awareness that all seven types of intelligence are equally important and your willingness to create a learning experience where participants can access them all.

The thirty-eight exercises in *Wellness 5* (as well as all others in the *Stress Management and Wellness Promotion* series), are designed to appeal to all seven ways of knowing. Almost all activate the *intrapersonal* dimension through individual reflection, and *interpersonal* dimension through a shared activity, group brainstorming, and/or sharing in pairs, small groups, or the large group.

Most of the longer processes, such as *Family Health Tree*(W5.150) and *Life Themes* (W5.151), typically use strategies that engage multiple intelligences. *Seven Ways of Knowing* (W5.162) is intended to explore each approach in depth. *Personal Vitality Kit* (W5.177) could easily be expanded to include multi-modal reminders of well-being. If you're trying to appeal to a certain mode of intelligence, try one of the following.

### ▧ VERBAL/LINGUISTIC
| | |
|---|---|
| *I See Myself* (W5.145c) | describing personal qualities |
| *Fact or Fiction* (W5.146) | reporting self-care behaviors |
| *Self-Esteem Pyramid* (W5.148) | verbalizing personal strengths |
| *Assertive Consumer* (W5.156) | complaint/commendation letters |
| *Take the Pledge* (W5.170) | paraphrasing a familiar commitment |
| *Ludicrous Workshops* (W5.175) | writing humorous course titles |
| *Strike Three* (W5.180) | storytelling/listening |

### ▧ LOGICAL/MATHEMATICAL
| | |
|---|---|
| *Anchors Aweigh* (W5.145a) | making analogies |
| *Health Transcript* (W5.147) | evaluating past performance |
| *TO DO Lists* (W5.149) | ranking priorities |
| *Family Health Tree* (W5.150) | ordering and classifying |
| *Pie Charts* (W5.152) | symbolic mathematical representation |

© 1995 Whole Person Press 210 W Michigan Duluth MN 55802      (800) 247-6789

Values and Self-Care (W5.155)            ranking, comparing, and contrasting
Relationship Report Card (W5.163)        checklist evaluation and comparison
If . . . Then (W5.167)                   cause and effect

▓ **VISUAL/SPATIAL**
Family Health Tree (W5.150)              genogram diagram
State Flag (W5.153)                      graphic representation of internal state
Mealtime Meditation (W5.157)             visualization of hungers
Imagery for a Healthy Heart (W5.159)     cardiovascular fitness visualization
Spiritual Fingerprint (W5.164)           artistic expression of inner truth
Self-Care Bouquet (W5.169)               affirmation drawing
Night Sky (W5.176)                       awe-inspiring visualization

▓ **BODY/KINESTHETIC**
Imaginary Ball Toss (W5.145b)            reinforce names with movement
Imagery for a Healthy Heart (W5.159)     explore circulatory system with imagery
Seventh Inning Stretch (W5.160)          memorable relaxation metaphors
Cleansing Breath (W5.172)                focused breathing for relaxation
For the Health of It (W5.173)            reinforce exercise through dance
Sights for Sore Eyes (W5.178)            soothing through touch
Stimulate & Integrate (W5.179)           sensory integration movements

▓ **MUSICAL/RHYTHMIC**
Anchors Aweigh (W5.145a)                 add the sound of your boat to intros
Spiritual Fingerprint (W5.164)           type of music may influence creations
Cleansing Breath (W5.172)                rhythmic yoga breathing
For the Health of It (W5.173)            music evokes body movement
Healthy Singalong (W5.174)               message in the music
Stimulate & Integrate (W5.179)           healthy rhythmic flow

▓ **INTRAPERSONAL**
Self-Esteem Pyramid (W5.148)             identify positive qualities in self
TO DO Lists (W5.149)                     explore personal goals
Life Themes (W5.151)                     discover recurring inner themes
Values and Self-Care (W5.155)            affirm motivating values
Mealtime Meditation (W5.157)             visualization to identify inner needs
Relationship Report Card (W5.163)        assess impact of others
Spiritual Fingerprint (W5.164)           get in touch with creative core
Leisure Pursuits (W5.165)                uncover primary motivators
Self-Care Bouquet (W5.169)               explore areas in need of support
Take the Pledge (W5.170)                 decide on resolutions for change

▓ **INTERPERSONAL**
All the Icebreakers engage participants in conversation and self-disclosure with
others. Most exercises in the Wellness Explorations, Self-Care, and Planning/
Closure sections involve some time in small group interaction, and these three focus
primarily on interpersonal knowing:

| | |
|---|---|
| *Mental Health Index* (W5.161) | group generates all the data |
| *Commercial Success* (W5.166) | collaborative creative effort |
| *Choose Wellness Anyway* (W5.171) | great show *of group solidarity* |

The principles of activating multiple intelligences are your invitation to new dimensions in training. Use this model to assess your strengths as a teacher, and then take up the creative challenge to activate all seven ways of knowing with every audience or subject matter.

To exercise your mental agility and push your boundaries a bit, take a self-care topic and use the suggestions on p. 82–83 in *Wellness 5* to imagine how you might approach the issue through each mode of intelligence. For example, if your topic were *vitamins*, you could ask participants to:

◆ **Verbal/Linguistic:** Create a poem or jump rope chant that extols the sources and virtues of different vitamins.

◆ **Logical/Mathematical:** Classify a group of vitamins in five different ways.

◆ **Visual/Spatial:** Make a diagram or poster to teach third graders (or senior citizens) about vitamins.

◆ **Body/Kinesthetic:** Create appropriate, memorable gestures for each vitamin, or make up a drama with people playing the roles of different vitamins.

◆ **Musical/Rhythmic:** Make up a sound and rhythm for your assigned vitamin and use it to teach others about its qualities.

◆ **Intrapersonal:** Write a personal statement: *If I could be a vitamin, which one would I be and why?*, or keep a journal of your week with vitamins.

◆ **Interpersonal:** In small groups, discuss the pros and cons of taking vitamin supplements, then develop a resolution on vitamins to be issued by the Surgeon General.

What we call creativity may be primarily the ability to exercise multiple intelligences and combine their power to solve problems—or present content material—in a new way.

Be adventurous.

© 1995 Whole Person Press 210 W Michigan Duluth MN 55802      (800) 247-6789

# 7
# Exercise
# Descriptions

This section includes a brief description of each exercise in the *Structured Exercises in Stress Management* and *Wellness Promotion* series, along with specific goals of the process and the time frame, organized by volume.

## STRESS 1                                              TABLE OF CONTENTS

© 1995 Whole Person Press 210 W Michigan Duluth MN 55802          (800) 247-6789

**8  THE JUGGLING ACT**                                   (40–60 min, p. 22)
In this novel stress assessment, participants inventory their stressors and recall the impact of stress on their internal and external environments.
  • *To identify stressors and assess personal stress level.*
  • *To explore the impact of stress on the body.*

**9  STRESSFUL OCCUPATIONS CONTEST**                      (35–45 min, p. 28)
Participants divide into occupational groups, brainstorm on-the-job stressors, and campaign to have theirs declared the "most stressful occupation." This lively exercise is particularly effective for mixed professional groups or in a setting that includes personnel from various job status levels.
  • *To explore the job-related stresses of various occupations.*
  • *To encourage creativity and humor.*

**10  STRESS RISK FACTORS**                               (10–20 min, p. 32)
In this assessment/chalktalk exercise participants reflect on their personal stress "at-risk-level" by examining their overall lifestyle patterns.
  • *To understand the long-term results of an overstressed, high-risk lifestyle.*
  • *To distinguish between those stressors you can control and those you cannot.*

**11  LIFETRAP 1: WORKAHOLISM**                           (60–90 min. p. 37)
This extended, multiprocess exercise allows participants to explore the meaning of work in their life. Participants check themselves against the symptoms of the "Hurry Sickness" that signals the onset of workaholism. They examine the results of this stress-laden lifestyle as well as the belief system that undergirds *Type A* behavior.
  • *To explore the meaning and place of work.*
  • *To identify the life-eroding stress bred by a lifestyle of work addiction.*
  • *To offer options for controlling and relieving the addiction to work.*

**12  THE AAAbc's OF STRESS MANAGEMENT**                  (45–60 min, p. 49)
This coping practicum teaches a simple paradigm for dealing with stress. Participants practice applying these strategies in role-play situations first and then apply the model to one of their own stressors.
  • *To explore alternatives for coping with stress.*
  • *To practice applying a coping model in hypothetical stressful situations.*
  • *To choose an effective stress management strategy for dealing with a specific personal stressor.*

**13  PROFESSIONAL SELF-CARE**                            (60 min, p. 56)
In this two-part exercise, participants first assess their personal and professional coping resources, then create a plan for minimizing stress in their work environment. The first part of the exercise makes a wonderful icebreaker.
  • *To reduce professionals' resistance to self-care strategies for dealing with stress.*
  • *To identify personal resources for stress management.*
  • *To explore the possible components of a work environment that maximizes energizers and minimizes stress exhaustion.*

**14  COPING SKILLS ASSESSMENT**                    (45–60 min, p. 63)
In this personal assessment process, participants explore their general coping skills and check out their skill level and usage pattern for twenty-one different coping techniques.
* *To assess and affirm stress management skills already in use.*
* *To identify target skills for future development of personal coping repertoire.*

**15  SKILL SKITS**                                    (60 min, p. 68)
This energizing and entertaining exercise fosters participants' creativity and *esprit de corps* while graphically illustrating the wide variety of coping alternatives available to all.
* *To explore a wide variety of coping strategies.*
* *To encourage creativity and high energy involvement in the learning process.*
* *To promote team-building.*

**16  STRESS BUFFER SHIELD**                        (20–30 min, p. 71)
Participants develop a personal stress buffer by affirming the qualities, life experiences, and coping skills that strengthen and protect them from negative stress. This process is especially effective as an icebreaker or closing affirmation.
* *To affirm personal qualities that buffer the effects of stress.*

**17  UNWINDING**                                    (20–30 min, p. 73)
Participants explore the stress-relaxation connection from both the academic and experiential perspectives in this revitalizing skill-builder.
* *To explore the relationship between stress and relaxation.*
* *To experience a state of profound relaxation.*

**18  I SURRENDER!**                                    (2–5 min, p. 78)
In three exercises that demonstrate surrender as a coping skill, participants launch a paper ship (**a. Goodbye**), practice passivity (**b. The Allowing Attitude**), and pray for a slower pace (**c. Slow Me Down Lord**).
* *To reinforce the importance of "letting go" as a stress management strategy.*
* *To illustrate the mind/body/spirit connection.*

**19  HUMOROUS INTERLUDES**                          (5–10 min, p. 82)
In this coping practicum collection, participants use music (**a. The Best Medicine**), a movie (**b. Beloved Husband of Irma**), and their imaginations (**c. Flight of Fancy**) to practice generating the healing power of laughter.
* *To explore laughter as a coping skill.*
* *To experience laughter as a tension reducer.*

**20  5–4–3–2–1 CONTACT**                            (20–30 min, p. 86)
In this energizing skill-builder, participants experiment with different styles of initiating contact with others.
* *To highlight the importance of interpersonal relationships as a stress management strategy.*
* *To experiment with different forms of making contact.*

© 1995 Whole Person Press 210 W Michigan Duluth MN 55802        (800) 247-6789

**21  GETTING OUT OF MY BOX**                        (60–90 min, p. 89)
In this reflective exercise, participants examine the chronically stressful sit-
uations in their lives and explore ways of caring for themselves in spite of the
painful life circumstances that may limit them.
  • *To recognize and label sources of chronic distress.*
  • *To make intentional choices about the situations that "box you in."*
  • *To experience the feeling of being lovable and acceptable in spite of
    personal limitations and chronic stressors.*

**22  ONE STEP AT A TIME**                           (20–30 min, p. 102)
This nine-part guide leads participants step-by-step through a creative plan-
ning process for coping with a stress-related problem.
  • *To subject at least one stress-related problem to a comprehensive planning
    approach.*
  • *To encourage creativity in action planning.*
  • *To elicit personal commitment to change.*

**23  POSTSCRIPT**                                   (15 min, p. 108)
In this action planning exercise, participants write themselves letters which
are then collected by the trainer and mailed sometime later as a reminder of
the learning that took place.
  • *To articulate and integrate stress management goals.*
  • *To provide a long-term link between the learning experience and the
    participants' daily living.*

**24  COPING SKILL AFFIRMATION**                     (60 min, p. 110)
This exercise is designed to affirm participants' positive stress management
coping skills, and is most effective at the conclusion of an ongoing learning
experience.
  • *To affirm positive coping skills in self and others.*
  • *To stimulate positive feedback and team building.*

**25  BOO-DOWN**                                     (5–8 min, p. 113)
This quick exercise exposes the role of irrational beliefs in creating stress and
actively engages the entire group in laughing at the stupidity of unreasonable
standards and expectations.
  • *To deal with irrational beliefs at a conscious, rather than unconscious level.*
  • *To demonstrate how beliefs can cause stress.*

**26  BREATH-LESS**                                  (2 min, p. 116)
A highly effective demonstration of stress and improper breathing.
  • *To demonstrate that under pressure most people forget to breathe deeply.*
  • *To provoke discussion about the importance of relaxation as a coping skill.*

**27  CATASTROPHE GAME**                             (10 min, p. 117)
Participants take turns exaggerating their stressful life situations into major
catastrophes, discovering in the process the absurdity of their "awfulizing"
habits.
  • *To highlight the assets and liabilities of complaining as a stress manage-
    ment technique.*

© 1995 Whole Person Press 210 W Michigan Duluth MN 55802          (800) 247-6789

**STRESS 2**                                                    **TABLE OF CONTENTS**

  • *To indicate that the toll of stress exhaustion is exacted on the whole person, not just the body.*

## 44  DRAGNET                                     (30–40 min, p. 28)
In this stress assessment, participants "unravel the mystery" of their stress by recording the facts and analyzing the clues they uncover.
  • *To identify current stressors.*
  • *To analyze the situational circumstances of stressors and to discover the common patterns that connect them.*

## 45  BACK TO THE DRAWING BOARD                    (50–75 min, p. 32)
In this major exercise, participants analyze the drainers and energizers of their work environment by drawing a symbolic picture of their work setting.
  • *To recognize factors in the job setting which produce distress.*
  • *To isolate factors in the job setting which nurture and reward.*
  • *To identify strategies for coping with organizational, work-related stress.*

## 46  LIFETRAP 2: HOOKED ON HELPING                (60–90 min, p. 36)
Participants affirm the admirable nature of their caring for others and also examine the long-term stress and resulting exhaustion that is inevitable when care-giving becomes an addiction. Although this extended, multi-process exercise is designed for "professional" helpers (nurses, counselors, clergy, teachers, etc), the issues apply to all caring people—especially working parents.
  • *To recognize, affirm, and rejoice in care-giving commitments.*
  • *To examine the stress that results when people get hooked on caring for others first, regardless of the cost to self.*
  • *To explore options for controlling the care-giver's addiction while still reaching out in caring commitments to others.*

## 47  CIRCUIT OVERLOAD                             (15–20 min, p. 46)
This assessment tool helps participants to see how much stress they are currently "loading on the circuits."
  • *To generate a personal and group list of stressors.*
  • *To explore the underlying causes of stress.*

## 48  I'VE GOT RHYTHM                              (15–20 min, p. 49)
This simple stress management strategy is based on the concept that there's a "right" time for everything. Participants identify the current rhythm of their lives and decide what plans will help them flow with, rather than fight against their natural rhythm.
  • *To illustrate that in stress management, attention to personal timing issues is important.*
  • *To identify and act upon current personal life rhythms.*

## 49  PILEUP COPERS                                (60 min, p. 54)
Using a unique deck of coping cards from the game "PILEUP" participants gain an overall view of possible coping options and identify their personal coping style, by sorting and discussing both the negative and positive coping cards.
  • *To illustrate the difference between positive and negative copers.*
  • *To explore the full range of coping options, and assess personal coping patterns.*

© 1995 Whole Person Press 210 W Michigan Duluth MN 55802      (800) 247-6789

**50  MONTH OF FUNDAYS**                              (20–30 min, p. 61)
Participants explore the power of play as a stress management resource and make a plan for incorporating play into their lifestyle every day of the coming month.
  • *To promote playfulness as a stress management technique.*
  • *To build play into each day's schedule for one month.*

**51  THE WORRY STOPPER**                             (30–40 min, p. 64)
In this thought-provoking chalktalk and assessment, participants use the criteria of control and importance to determine what's worth worrying about.
  • *To explore the multitudes of things people worry about—both the trivial and the important.*
  • *To underline the importance of values in effective stress management.*
  • *To learn a tool for deciding what's worth worrying about.*

**52  CONSULTANTS UNLIMITED**                         (30–40 min, p. 70)
Participants act as a consultation team engaged to devise alternative strategies for managing each others' "on-the-job" stressors.
  • *To generate and evaluate coping strategies for specific job stressors.*
  • *To reinforce the concept of peer consultation as a problem-solving model.*

**53  ATTITUDE ADJUSTMENT HOUR**                      (25–35 min, p. 73)
In this lively exercise, participants practice the art of altering their viewpoint by telling and retelling the stories of their day from different perspectives.
  • *To demonstrate the role of perception in the management of stress.*
  • *To practice making conscious shifts in perpetual patterns.*

**54  SPEAK UP!**                                     (40–45 min, p. 77)
Participants explore the value of assertiveness as a coping skill by pairing up and experimenting with alternative styles both for making requests and for saying "no."
  • *To assess personal comfort and skill in asking for things and in saying no.*
  • *To learn the difference between effective and ineffective requests and refusals and practice assertive, direct expression of requests and refusals.*

**55  AFFIRMATIVE ACTION PLAN**                       (40–50 min, p. 81)
In this attitude-changing exercise, participants draw up a plan for using affirmation to manage a workplace stressor.
  • *To explore the potential of affirmation as a stress management skill.*
  • *To increase participants' repertoire of affirming behaviors.*
  • *To develop on-the-job applications for affirmation skills.*

**56  ANCHORING**                                     (30 min, p. 88)
Participants guide one another through a relaxation fantasy and "anchor" the comfortable feelings they experience for later recall and stimulation of the relaxation response.
  • *To develop a quick self-eliciting resource for relaxation.*
  • *To demonstrate the potency of recalled experience in evoking relaxation responses.*

**57  THE ABC'S OF TIME**                                    (40–50 min, p. 92)
This skill-building exercise illustrates the importance of spending time where
it counts. Participants list the activities and tasks that consumed yesterday's
24 hours, then assess whether or not they invested effort in their top priorities.
  • *To analyze time use patterns.*
  • *To distinguish the "A" priorities from the "B" and "C" tasks.*
  • *To understand and practice the major time management skills.*

**58  PERSONAL/PROFESSIONAL REVIEW**              (10–15 min, p. 97)
Participants review the session and affirm what they have gained from the
learning experience.
  • *To apply concepts to real life situations.*
  • *To end the session on a positive note.*

**59  MANAGER OF THE YEAR**                             (45–60 min, p. 98)
In this closing affirmation,,, participants write recommendations for them-
selves and campaign for "Stress Manager of the Year" awards.
  • *To enhance self-perceptions of competence for dealing with stress.*
  • *To provide closure for the learning experience.*
  • *To promote feedback among participants.*

**60  GOALS, OBSTACLES AND ACTIONS**             (60 min, p. 102)
This in-depth planning exercise helps participants set goals, formulate strat-
egies for moving toward their goals, and monitor their progress.
  • *To identify a limited number of specific behavior-changing goals.*
  • *To formulate a plan of action for overcoming the obstacles that hold you
    back, and to monitor your step-by-step progress toward your goals.*

**61  25 WORDS OR LESS**                                 (10–15 min, p. 108)
Participants exchange advice for managing stress.
  • *To articulate what was learned about stress management.*
  • *To add drama, suspense, and energy to the transfer-of-learning process.*

**62  STRESS AND COPING JOURNAL**                (5–10 min, p. 110)
This on-going homework assignment helps participants monitor their stress
and apply the management techniques learned during a several week course.
(three 15–30 minute homework periods)
  • *To apply concepts to real-life situations.*
  • *To monitor stress levels and progress in implementation of coping skills.*

**63  THE GARDEN**                                       (5 min, p. 113)
This poignant parable focuses on the difference between "play" and "scor-
ing."
  • *To reflect on the purpose of life, interactions with others, and play.*

**64  HAND-TO-HAND CONTACT**                       (10 min, p. 115)
In this soothing relaxation break, participants trade hand massages.
  • *To reduce tension in fingers and hands.*
  • *To learn nonthreatening massage techniques.*

© 1995 Whole Person Press 210 W Michigan Duluth MN 55802      (800) 247-6789

**65  HELPERS ANONYMOUS**                                    (5 min, p. 118)
In this tongue-in-cheek initiation rite, participants confess their addiction to helping and learning the HA theme song.
  • *To poke fun at a typical stress-producing habit.*
  • *To affirm that personal wants and needs are important.*

**66  MUSICAL MOVEMENT**                                    (10–15 min, p. 120)
A montage of musical styles provides the background and beat for tension-reducing interpretive movement.
  • *To expand awareness of the value of music and movement as coping techniques.*
  • *To provide a playful interlude.*

**67  ROUND OF APPLAUSE**                                    (2 min, p. 122)
In this hand-warming and heartwarming energizer, participants applaud their accomplishments and give each other a standing ovation.
  • *To promote affirmation as a stress management strategy.*
  • *To boost group energy.*

**68  SEAWEED AND OAK**                                    (5–10 min, p. 123)
Participants alter their energy flow, using fantasy to become as flexible as floating seaweed and as sturdy as an oak tree.
  • *To become aware of how thoughts and energy flow are interrelated.*
  • *To compare spontaneity and control in two contrasting experiences of relaxation.*

**69  STRESS STRETCHERS**                                    (5–10 min, p. 125)
Rubberbands illustrate the tension/relaxation dynamics of stress and demonstrate the need for creativity in coping.
  • *To illustrate the individuality of healthy stress and tension levels.*
  • *To get the creative juices flowing and relieve the tension of talking about stress.*

**70  TARGET PRACTICE**                                    (10 min, p. 127)
Participants choose a coping skill and experiment with using it during a coffee or lunch break.
  • *To visualize where, when, and how a specific stress management strategy might be useful.*
  • *To practice a new or under-utilized coping skill.*

**71  TEN-SECOND BREAK**                                    (5 min, p. 129)
Participants learn a ten-second breathing and autosuggestion break that's ideal for instant stress relief.
  • *To interrupt or prevent tension buildup.*

**72  TREASURE CHEST**                                    (15–20 min, p. 131)
In this colorful guided fantasy, participants discover a treasure chest containing a "gift" they need.
  • *To synthesize and "own" what has been learned during the session.*

---

## STRESS 3                                                    TABLE OF CONTENTS

© 1995 Whole Person Press 210 W Michigan Duluth MN 55802          (800) 247-6789

**80  ON THE SPOT**                                       (30–60 min, p. 21)

In this thought-provoking process, participants examine situations in which they are most vulnerable to manipulations, and using *Ten Steps to Critical Thinking,* brainstorm ways to avoid being manipulated in the future.

  • *To increase awareness of the stress of manipulation.*
  • *To apply critical thinking techniques as a stress management strategy in potentially manipulative situations.*

**81  DRAINERS AND ENERGIZERS**                         (10–25 min, p. 26)

The checklists used in this exercise prompt participants to identify the negative stressors in their lives that drain them, as well as the positive energizers that refill them—at work, at home, and at play.

  • *To identify the daily drainers that deplete energy.*
  • *To recognize and utilize the daily energizers that restore vitality.*

**82  LIFETRAP 3: SICK OF CHANGE**                      (60–90 min, p. 30)

In this multiphase exercise, participants examine the role of change in their lives and the stress it creates. The double assessment, both objective and subjective, allows them ample opportunity to explore their current risk level and to articulate with each other the nature of the changes they are experiencing. Finally, participants plan strategies for taking charge of their own level and pace of change as they move into the future.

  • *To understand the connection between stress, life changes, and health.*
  • *To assess the levels and types of change present in current life situations.*
  • *To explore strategies for managing the stress of change.*

**83  JOB DESCRIPTIONS**                                    (60 min, p. 40)

Participants divide into gender groups to examine how sex role stereotyping can lead to the interpersonal stress of conflicting expectations.

  • *To demonstrate role conflict as a source of stress.*
  • *To study role stereotypes that can cause stress and interfere with interpersonal communication.*
  • *To apply attitude awareness as a technique in stress management.*

**84  THE LAST CHRISTMAS TREE**                         (20–30 min, p. 44)

This fantasy exercise enables participants to explore the stress associated with rejection.

  • *To identify the stress of actual or potential rejection.*
  • *To discover alternative perceptions of the rejection experience.*

**85  METAPHORS**                                        (40–50 min, p. 49)

Participants study the form and function of various objects, seeking clues to creative stress management.

  • *To provide a model for back-home problem solving.*
  • *To promote creativity and nonlinear approaches to stress management.*

**86  S.O.S. FOR STRESS**                                (30–50 min, p. 54)

Participants learn an overarching paradigm for coping with stress and apply the specific strategies from this model to a personal stressor of their choice.

  • *To expand awareness of multiple coping options for any single stressor.*
  • *To activate under-utilized or neglected skills for managing stress.*

**87  STRESS CLUSTERS CLINIC**                    (40–60 min, p. 59)
In this challenging card game participants utilize separate decks of stressor cards and coping cards to create stress scenarios and strategies for coping based on "the luck of the draw."
- *To explore the stress generated by clusters of change.*
- *To apply specific coping skills to a lifelike stress scenario.*
- *To promote problem-solving approaches to coping with stress.*

**88  CORPORATE PRESENTATION**                    (20–30 min, p. 66)
In this affirming small group activity, participants give themselves a lecture about the ten best methods for managing stress.
- *To pool wisdom about coping with stress.*
- *To provide an overview of stress management strategies.*

**89  IMAGINE SUCCESS**                           (15–30 min, p. 68)
Participants practice the technique of positive visualization, imagining themselves as successfully employing a selected coping skill.
- *To apply a practical principle of successful stress management within the learning experience.*
- *To experience the power of postive visualization.*

**90  CONFLICT MANAGEMENT**                       (60 min, p. 73)
In this thought-provoking learning experience participants explore four conflict-prevention skills and experiment with applying them to specific conflict situations.
- *To identify conflict situations that cause stress.*
- *To discover and practice alternative approaches for preventing or managing conflict.*

**91  EIGHT-MINUTE STRESS BREAK**                 (10 min, p. 80)
Participants learn a 15-step stretch routine that can be used as a stress break any time of the day.
- *To demonstrate the effectiveness of exercise as a stress management technique.*
- *To stretch all the major muscle groups.*

**92  STOP LOOK AND LISTEN**                      (60 min, p. 84)
Using a do-it-yourself study guide, trios of participants experiment with techniques to improve listening skills and explore applications of empathy as a stress management strategy.
- *To explore the value of listening as a coping skill in stressful situations.*
- *To practice listening skills.*

**93  CENTERING MEDITATION**                      (25–40 min, p. 92)
Participants experience the quieting process of meditation and the focusing power of visualization in this guided fantasy.
- *To learn the principles of meditation and imagery as skills for relaxation.*
- *To experience quiet, calm, peace, and a sense of inner vision.*

---

© 1995 Whole Person Press 210 W Michigan Duluth MN 55802          (800) 247-6789

**94  CLOSING FORMATION**                                    (10–30 min, p. 97)
In this round-robin ending, participants pair up with many different partners to
briefly share reactions, insights, and coping plans.
* *To review highlights of the learning experience and solidify specific plans
  for better stress management.*
* *To touch base with many other participants before ending the session/
  course.*

**95  EXIT INTERVIEW**                                       (20–30 min, p. 100)
In dyads, participants review course content and publicly affirm their plans for
improved stress management.
* *To provide closure and reinforce concepts and techniques presented during the learning experience.*
* *To articulate plans for integrating and implementing stress management
  principles in daily life.*

**96  RECIPE FOR SUCCESS WITH STRESS**                       (25–30 min, p. 104)
Participants reflect on the ingredients for successful stress management as
they cook up innovative personal recipes for handling stress.
* *To review qualities that are particularly effective in coping with stress.*
* *To promote creativity, humor, and self-expression.*

**97  MY STRESS REDUCTION PROGRAM**                          (20–30 min, p. 107)
This step-by-step planning process helps participants formulate a specific
plan for managing a stress-related problem.
* *To practice a process for developing a stress management program
  tailored to deal with specific stressors.*
* *To elicit personal commitment to change.*

**98  CHANGE PENTAGON**                                      (15–30 min, p. 110)
Participants explore each aspect of life (mental, physical, interpersonal,
spiritual, and lifestyle) seeking positive alternatives for managing stress. They
then draw up a "whole person" plan for dealing with specific problem situations.
* *To isolate stressful situations that require attention.*
* *To expand awareness of coping options and make a plan for coping in a
  new way with a stressful situation.*

**99  KICKING YOUR STRESS CAN-CAN**                          (5 min, p. 113)
Participants kick up their heels as they symbolically kick sources of stress out
of their lives.
* *To demonstrate exercise as a pleasurable and effective stress-reducer.*
* *To target specific stressors for change.*

**100  CHINESE SWING**                                       (10 min, p. 114)
In this invigorating exercise break, participants learn an ancient oriental tech-
nique for releasing stress.
* *To stimulate energy flow in the body and to promote deep breathing.*
* *To discharge muscular tension.*

**101  CLOUDS TO SUNSHINE**                            (3–5 min, p. 116)
This adaptation of a traditional t'ai chi exercise allows participants to breathe and stretch easily while imagining four different scenes from nature.
* *To focus attention and let go of mental distractions.*
* *To stretch and release tension from the muscles in the arms and back.*

**102  CREATE A SINGALONG**                            (10–15 min, p. 118)
Participants compose stress and coping lyrics for familiar melodies and then perform their "work" or the group.
* *To reinforce concepts taught in the session or course.*
* *To promote group creativity and spontaneity.*

**103  GROANS AND MOANS**                              (5–15 min, p. 120)
In this noisy energizer, participants experiment with an old-fashioned remedy for stress.
* *To demonstrate the effectiveness of groaning as a tension-relieving technique.*
* *To relax and let go.*

**104  TUG OF WAR**                                    (5–10 min, p. 122)
In this game of strategy, participants pair up to explore alternative approaches to conflict.
* *To visually explore personal styles of approaching conflict.*

**105  WARM HANDS**                                    (5–10 min, p. 124)
In this brief introduction to the potential of autogenics, participants imagine their way to warm hands and a profound sense of relaxation.
* *To demonstrate the power of autogenic-like techniques for relaxation.*

**106  WHAT'S THE HURRY?**                             (5 min, p. 126)
This touching parable points out how striving too hard to reach a goal may have stressful side effects.
* *To help participants reflect on the potential risks of Type A behavior.*

**107  YOU'RE NOT LISTENING!**                         (5–10 min, p. 129)
In this riotous energizer, partners work hard at "not listening" to each other and then brainstorm essentials of good listening.
* *To identify key elements of effective listening.*
* *To promote group interaction and playfulness.*

**108  PUSHING MY BUTTONS**                            (10–15 min, p. 131)
In this unusual self-care break, participants stimulate several acupressure points to get their energy flowing again.
* *To introduce the concept of energy flow.*
* *To energize and revitalize the group.*

© 1995 Whole Person Press 210 W Michigan Duluth MN 55802          (800) 247-6789

## STRESS 4                                          TABLE OF CONTENTS

*To expand awareness of interventions for reducing physical stress.*

**117 ON THE JOB STRESS GRID**                    (25–40 min, p. 25)
Participants use a special grid to pinpoint their job stress and its sources, then rank the intensity of their stress, identify their job "hot spots," and explore possibilities for coping.
- *To identify the variety and intensity of vocation-related stressors.*
- *To seek methods of coping with job-related "hot spots" that could lead to burnout.*

**118 STRESS ATTITUDES SURVEY**                   (20–30 min, p. 33)
Participants use their feet and heads to express and explore attitudes toward stress in this human values continuum.
- *To raise consciousness about personal beliefs related to stress.*
- *To reevaluate and articulate attitudes toward stress.*
- *To promote group interaction and involvement.*

**119 STRESS SKETCH**                             (30–40 min, p. 37)
In this imaginative stress assessment, participants draw a major life stress and engage it in a provocative conversation.
- *To explore in depth the mind/body/spirit dimensions of a major life struggle.*
- *To encourage nonlinear approaches to stress management.*
- *To affirm individuals' capacity for insight into the source and impact of stress in their lives.*

**120 LIFETRAP 4: GOOD GRIEF?**                   (60–90 min, p. 41)
In this powerful self-reflection and sharing exercise, participants explore loss as a common source of stress, and grieving as a natural process of healing. They identify distressing symptoms of a personal loss, compare their experience with the typical stages of grief, and explore methods for reducing the stress of grief.
- *To recognize that while every loss causes distress, healthy grieving leads toward healing.*
- *To identify the normal stages of the grief process.*
- *To foster healthful skills for coping with the pain of loss.*

**121 A GOOD STRESS MANAGER**                     (30–60 min, p. 49)
In this two-stage exercise, participants brainstorm qualities and behaviors of effective stress managers, then in small groups compile their own coping assessment instruments and test themselves.
- *To identify effective attitudes and approaches for managing stress.*
- *To elicit and reinforce participants' internal wisdom.*
- *To assess personal coping style.*

**122 OBLIGATION OVERLOAD**                       (45 min, p. 56)
Participants envision reducing their stress by eliminating specific obligations, then in small groups practice standing up to internal and external pressures that make such a change difficult.
- *To understand the many factors that keep us overcommitted.*
- *To practice standing up to pressure from outside and pressure from within when attempting to make a change.*

---

© 1995 Whole Person Press 210 W Michigan Duluth MN 55802        (800) 247-6789

**123  METAPHORS 2**                                        (20–30 min, p. 61)
In this imagination-stretching process, participants uncover new approaches to a stressful situation.
* *To promote creative approaches to stress management.*
* *To view a current stressful situation from a new perspective that suggests alternatives for coping.*

**124  911 EMERGENCY PLAN**                                 (20–30 min, p. 65)
In this exploration of coping in crisis situations, participants develop a personalized strategy for emergency stress management.
* *To explore options for coping in acutely stressful situations.*
* *To develop a personal strategy for managing stress in a crisis.*

**125  REST IN PEACE**                                      (15–20 min, p. 68)
In this unusual visualization, participants lay to rest negative attitudes, perceptions, and patterns that cause them stress.
* *To identify adaptive patterns that have outlived their usefulness.*
* *To practice a technique for letting go of stress.*

**126  GO FOR THE GOLD**                                    (30–40 min, p. 73)
In this skill-building exercise, participants examine their personal goal-setting process and explore the effectiveness of organizing their day-to-day decisions toward specific, targeted goals.
* *To assess current levels of personal planning.*
* *To illustrate the benefits of regular goal-setting.*
* *To facilitate the development of positive habits and skills that help individuals be productive and reach personal targets.*

**127  SHIFTING GEARS**                                     (15–30 min, p. 82)
In this lively skill builder, participants learn specific techniques to manage stress once they've recognized situations in which they need to slow down, "rev" up, or loosen up.
* *To recognize body/mind/spirit signals that indicate the need for a change of pace.*
* *To explore changing tempo as a vital stress management skill.*

**128  OPEN UP**                                            (30–40 min, p. 87)
Participants use a paper bag to explore the potential of self-disclosure as a stress management technique and generate a list of helpful "ears" for coping with tough times.
* *To experience the benefits of talking about stress as an effective coping technique.*
* *To practice self-disclosure.*
* *To raise consciousness about resources for help in managing stress.*

**129  BIOFEEDBACK**                                        (20–25 min, p. 92)
Participants use miniature thermometers to monitor fluctuating stress levels as they practice a simple relaxation routine.
* *To explore the role of self-monitoring (biofeedback) as an essential skill in stress management.*

• *To practice an effective relaxation technique.*

**130  ABCDEFG PLANNER**                          (20–30 min, p. 97)
Participants use a seven-step process to devise a concrete plan for managing one life stressor more effectively.
• *To learn and apply a systematic planning process.*
• *To elicit personal commitment to change.*

**131  SO WHAT?**                                (10–15 min, p. 102)
This quick and easy planner challenges participants to summarize what they have learned and apply it in concrete ways to their life situations.
• *To review the key concepts from the learning experience.*
• *To articulate possibilities and plans for implementing stress management principles in daily life.*

**132  GROUP BANNER**                            (15–25 min, p. 105)
In small groups, participants use the contents of a grab bag to create graphic tributes to what they have learned.
• *To review and affirm insights from the learning experience.*
• *To build camaraderie and group spirit.*
• *To provide a playful/creative counterpoint to more serious subject matter.*

**133  PAT ON THE BACK**                         (20–30 min, p. 107)
Participants use the colorful PILEUP card game to affirm stress management skills, in themselves and each other.
• *To review the wide variety of options possible for managing stress.*
• *To affirm positive coping efforts.*
• *To provide closure.*

**134  DEAR ME P.S.**                            (10–15 min, p. 112)
This closing/evaluation tool helps participants reflect on what they have learned and focus on potential applications.
• *To conceptualize, articulate, and apply learning.*

**135  GIRAFFE**                                 (5 min, p. 113)
In this pleasurable visualization, participants learn a simple stretch routine for relaxing the neck and shoulders.
• *To relieve tension in the muscles of the neck and shoulders.*

**136  HOT TUB**                                 (8 min, p. 115)
In this unusual relaxation experience, participants unwind in the soothing warmth of an imaginary hot springs.
• *To provide an **in vivo** relaxation experience.*
• *To demonstrate the power of visualization as a tension-reduction strategy.*

**137  HOW TO SWIM WITH SHARKS**                 (5 min, p. 118)
This perceptive parody offers humorous advice for dealing with hostile workplace environments.
• *To explore the stress of dealing with hostile people in difficult situations.*
• *To illustrate that at times self-defense may be the best—or only—strategy.*

© 1995 Whole Person Press 210 W Michigan Duluth MN 55802          (800) 247-6789

**138  HUMAN KNOTS**                                    (5–10 min, p. 120)
In this group imbroglio, participants learn firsthand how to unwind when they're
tied up in knots.
  • *To demonstrate that it takes effort to reverse the accumulation of tension
    that accompanies stress.*

**139  MERRY-GO-ROUND**                                 (5–15 min, p. 122)
In this rowdy energizer, participants discover the stress of taking on too many
burdens.
  • *To demonstrate the strain of accumulated stress.*
  • *To experience physical and emotional symptoms of stress.*

**140  MICROWAVE**                                      (2 min, p. 124)
In this invigorating stretch break for large groups, participants join in a familiar
grandstand sport.
  • *To provide an energizing break for participants.*
  • *To stretch and release accumulated tension.*

**141  THE MUSTARD SEED**                               (5 min, p. 126)
This parable poignantly illustrates that loss and death are inescapable part-
ners with life.
  • *To illustrate that no one is immune from grief.*
  • *To affirm that those who grow do so not by avoiding death, but by em-
    bracing it.*

**142  REVITALIZE YOUR EYES**                           (2–5 min each, p. 128)
In this ancient self-care break, participants practice acupressure techniques
for relieving tension and strain in a busy body part.
  • *To learn strategies for reducing eyestrain and tension.*

**143  SIGH OF RELIEF**                                 (3–5 minutes, p. 130)
This quick energizer provides an expressive relaxation break.
  • *To release accumulated tension.*
  • *To increase participants' repertoire of instant stress relievers.*

**144  SNAP, CRACKLE, POP**                             (5–10 min, p. 132)
Participants join forces to get their blood moving in this body clapping stress
break.
  • *To relieve tension.*
  • *To promote interaction and energize the group.*

**STRESS 5**                                          **TABLE OF CONTENTS**

© 1995 Whole Person Press 210 W Michigan Duluth MN 55802          (800) 247-6789

 • *To develop tools for raising self-esteem.*
 • *To empower women to take actions to reduce their stress.*

**153  PICK YOUR BATTLES**                                    (30 min, p. 34)
This systematic procedure, which helps participants target stressors that are important to change, is especially useful when stress is overwhelming or it's difficult to decide where to start.
 • *To identify sources of stress.*
 • *To rank stressors in relation to their personal impact, potential for change, and relevance or priority.*

**154  STORMY PASSAGES**                                    (20–30 min, p. 38)
In this open-ended stress assessment, participants visualize their reactions to a thunderstorm and apply their insight to the stormy passages of life.
 • *To identify stressful life situations and habitual coping patterns.*
 • *To activate emotional resources as motivators for insight and change.*

**155  WINDOWS ON STRESS**                                    (30–45 min, p. 43)
In this adaptable, multilayered assessment, participants use mental software to explore the interactive windows of their stress.
 • *To explore the multifaceted nature of a stress that needs attention.*
 • *To break down a complex life stress into more manageable components.*

**156  MANAGING JOB STRESS**                                    (20–60 min, p. 49)
This thought-provoking short video and self-analysis process gives participants the tools they need to identify, analyze, and plan strategies for coping with on-the-job stress.
 • *To recognize the variety and intensity of work-related stresses.*
 • *To learn new skills and ways of coping with "hot spots" that cause job stress.*

**157  QUESTIONABLE COPERS**                                    (30–40 min, p. 51)
Participants analyze their negative coping patterns and explore healthier alternatives.
 • *To identify questionable coping strategies and typical stressful situations where they are used.*
 • *To track occurrences of negative coping behaviors and substitute more positive strategies.*

**158  SILVER LININGS**                                    (20–30 min, p. 55)
In this thoughtful exercise, participants discover silver linings in a problem-cloud and use these ribbons of light as inspiration for coping strategies.
 • *To discover opportunities for growth inherent in a problem.*
 • *To develop strategies for handling a troublesome dilemma.*

**159  STRESS MANAGEMENT ALPHABET**                                    (50–60 min, p. 59)
This widely acclaimed prescription for stress management is as simple as ABC, fun to do, and exciting to learn.
 • *To learn a new paradigm for managing stress.*
 • *To apply stress management strategies to personal life situations.*

**160  YESTERDAY, TODAY, AND TOMORROW**          (20–30 min, p. 66)
In this empowering exercise, participants assess the amount of time they mentally spend in the past, present, and future, and are encouraged to capitalize on the power of the present moment.
  • *To understand how being present to ourselves keeps us well.*
  • *To learn practical ideas for staying in the present moment.*

**161  AFFIRMATION CALENDAR**                     (25–30 min, p. 71)
Participants fill a calendar with rich, positive statements about themselves, and read these thoughts for daily affirmations in the coming month.
  • *To affirm positive attitudes and behaviors.*
  • *To practice affirmation as a stress management skill.*

**162  EATING UNDER STRESS**                      (40–45 min, p. 76)
Participants examine their patterns of eating, drinking, and smoking under stress, and develop strategies for modifying problem behaviors.
  • *To identify personal patterns of eating, drinking, or smoking under stress.*
  • *To learn more positive strategies for managing these stress symptoms.*

**163  KEEP YOUR COOL**                           (60–90 min, p. 81)
This action-oriented exercise allows participants to practice skills for managing anger in provocative situations.
  • *To identify positive and negative effects of anger.*
  • *To minimize the negative effects of anger and maximize the positive effects.*
  • *To develop alternative strategies for dealing with angry feelings.*

**164  REMOTE CONTROL**                           (20–30 min, p. 91)
In this empowering exercise, participants draw upon innate, natural skills to change their mood and direct their behavior.
  • *To recognize that we can control our thoughts, feelings, and actions.*
  • *To reduce stress by actively changing our thought patterns.*

**165  YOGA**                                     (30–60 min, p. 94)
Participants experiment with basic breathing and posture techniques in this exploration of the stress management benefits of yoga.
  • *To explore the philosophy and techniques of yoga.*
  • *To reduce tension and increase mental clarity.*

**166  FIVE AND TEN**                             (10–15 min, p. 99)
In this quick assessment and planning process, participants focus on five stressors and a ten-step strategy for coping with one.
  • *To develop a plan of action to deal with a troublesome stressor.*

**167  GO FLY A KITE**                            (10–20 min, p. 101)
In this uplifting ending to a learning experience, participants create a personal stress management program that is guaranteed to fly.
  • *To identify stressful feelings, attitudes, and behaviors as targets for change.*
  • *To reaffirm uplifting personal qualities and coping skills.*

© 1995 Whole Person Press 210 W Michigan Duluth MN 55802          (800) 247-6789

**168  HOPE CHEST**                                         (15–20 min, p. 105)
Participants fill their chests with all their hopes for change in this thoughtful, upbeat exercise.
  • *To identify goals for change.*
  • *To plan for ways to accomplish these goals.*

**169  KEY LEARNING**                                       (5–10 min, p. 108)
In this simple, effective process for closure and planning, participants write important insights and personal applications on three keys which will open the door for change.
  • *To summarize learning and apply ideas to current life situations.*

**170  STRESS EXAMINER**                                    (20–30 min, p. 111)
In this creative, playful exercise, participants imagine the contents of a stress management newspaper that provides exactly the kind of information they need.
  • *To summarize learnings about stress management.*
  • *To identify resources needed for personal change.*

**171  ANTI-STRESS COFFEE BREAK**                           (10–15 min, p. 113)
Participants fill their tanks with energizing foods and beverages, instead of stress foods like caffeine and sugars.
  • *To provide participants with foods which nourish their bodies and restore feelings of vitality.*

**172  BREATH PRAYER**                                      (8–10 min, p. 115)
Participants tap into their inner healing resources in this relaxing, rhythmic affirmation/meditation.
  • *To provide relaxation and centering.*
  • *To identify and affirm core truths.*

**173  COBRA**                                              (5 min, p. 118)
This gentle yoga movement stretches the back muscles, expands the chest, and stimulates the inner organs.
  • *To reduce tension and release trapped energy.*
  • *To promote flexibility and resiliency.*

**174  HAND DANCING**                                       (10 min, p. 120)
Even those who hate to dance will love this playful, easy process for mimicking a partner's hand movements to music.
  • *To get energized and feel connected to other group members.*
  • *To explore issues of control.*

**175  HUMMING BREATH**                                     (3–5 min, p. 122)
Participants enjoy a relaxing internal massage as they practice a mystical, musical yoga technique for reducing tension.
  • *To relax and get centered.*
  • *To experiment with an alternative technique for coping with stress.*

**176  STRESS SQUEEZERS**                                    (10–15 min, p. 124)
In this humorous activity, participants reflect on their stress levels and coping styles as they sculpt a personalized desktop stress reducer.
- *To identify life stressors.*
- *To explore symbolic and physical tension relief.*

**177  SUPERMAN**                                            (5–10 min, p. 126)
In this tongue-in-cheek discussion of performance and perfectionism, men and women are challenged to accept their imperfections and learn from their mistakes.
- *To put failures into perspective.*

**178  TOO BAD!**                                            (10–15 min, p. 129)
Participants poke gentle fun at themselves and each other by taking turns complaining and sympathizing about life's minor hassles.
- *To learn not to take problems too seriously.*
- *To shift from a complaining mode to a coping mode.*

**179  TROUBLE BUBBLES**                                     (5–10 min, p. 131)
This short visualization allows participants to get rid of negative feelings by imagining them as bubbles that they blow away.
- *To let go of stressful thoughts and feelings.*

**180  TRY, TRY AGAIN**                                      (5 min, p. 133)
This surprising parable underlines the importance of developing a wide repertoire of coping strategies for managing stress.
- *To reinforce new problem-solving skills.*
- *To poke fun at people's propensity for intensity.*

© 1995 Whole Person Press 210 W Michigan Duluth MN 55802          (800) 247-6789

## WELLNESS 1                                         TABLE OF CONTENTS

**8  VITALITY FACTORS**                                        (30–45 min, p. 25)
This exercise allows individuals to assess their strengths and weaknesses in unique areas of high vitality (eg, body maintenance, letting go, celebrating, etc).
  • *To identify personal vitality factors and potential areas of revitalization.*
  • *To provide structure and motivation for lifestyle changes.*

**9  WELLNESS CONGRESS**                                       (90–120 min, p. 30)
This exercise opens up for participants the wide range of issues and factors to be considered as part of health and wellness by challenging participants to formulate and adopt a group creed of wellness.
  • *To help participants recognize their own beliefs and biases.*
  • *To stimulate spirited discussion regarding the qualities of whole person health and their relative importance.*

**10  HEALTH/ILLNESS IMAGES**                                  (90 min, p. 38)
This extended reflection exercise helps participants recognize the ebb and flow of sickness and health in their lives and uncover personal symbols that shape their lifestyle patterns.
  • *To recognize the patterns of health and illness exhibited over a lifetime.*
  • *To identify the major symbols and life scripts that drive lifestyle decision-making.*
  • *To foster more conscious decision-making for self-care.*

**11  THE MARATHON STRATEGY**                                 (15 min, p. 49)
This chalktalk utilizes the metaphor of a marathon to demonstrate that over the "long run" those who care for themselves and take time to stop and fill up along the way finish the race with gusto to spare.
  • *To explore the importance of nourishment throughout life.*
  • *To identify personal energizers for refreshment.*

**12  DAILY RITUALS**                                          (10–15 min, p. 54)
This short exercise helps participants identify and rate their small daily rituals that accompany wake-up time, lunchtime, dinner/evening-time, and bedtime.
  • *To highlight personal awareness of daily patterns.*
  • *To identify a surefire energizer for each period of the day.*

**13  LETTER FROM THE INTERIOR**                              (20–30 min, p. 56)
Participants explore the impact of physical self-care practices by writing a letter from their body detailing all of its complaints and commendations.
  • *To heighten awareness of physical self-care patterns and their impact on well-being.*
  • *To target specific negative self-care habits that need modification.*
  • *To reinforce positive self-care practices.*

**14  THE LAST MEAL**                                          (15–30 min, p. 58)
Participants record and analyze the quality and quantity consumed at their last meal.
  • *To highlight participants' eating patterns and their effects.*
  • *To provoke a discussion of positive nutrition habits.*

© 1995 Whole Person Press 210 W Michigan Duluth MN 55802          (800) 247-6789

**15  THE EXERCISE EXERCISE**                              (15 min, p. 62)
This short group exercise routine, complete from warm-up to cool down, will get the group "psyched" for learning.
- *To demonstrate the benefits of exercise—fun, exhilaration, and stress reduction.*
- *To rejuvenate participants.*
- *To learn target pulse monitoring of aerobic exercise.*

**16  SANCTUARY**                                        (15–30 min, p. 67)
This technique demonstrates the use of an imagery "sanctuary," or brief retreat from daily stresses.
- *To demonstrate the vivid and powerful effects of relaxing imagery.*
- *To develop a pleasant self-induced focus of attention for relaxation.*

**17  MARCO POLO**                                       (15–20 min, p. 70)
This thought-provoking short film and self-analysis process allows participants to explore the issue of mental health from the viewpoint of a young child.
- *To rediscover childlike qualities of mental health.*
- *To identify strategies for recapturing and increasing desired qualities.*

**18  DISCRIMINATING FEELER**                            (30–45 min, p. 74)
This exercise explores the importance of feelings in mental health, emotions that might be aroused in specific situations, and personal feeling preferences and patterns.
- *To expand your vocabulary of feeling words.*
- *To explore emotional responses to a variety of situations.*
- *To identify personal response styles and consider other options.*

**19  INTERPERSONAL NEEDS**                              (60–90 min, p. 81)
In this exercise, participants examine their social networks and analyze how well their interpersonal needs are being met.
- *To highlight the variety of intensity and purpose within relationships.*
- *To recognize interpersonal needs and to identify various sources of support.*
- *To motivate participants to be intentional in building a support network that nurtures them at many levels of need.*

**20  IRISH SWEEPSTAKES**                                (20–30 min, p. 90)
Participants plan a budget for their million dollar sweepstakes win and examine the implied values.
- *To foster creative daydreaming.*
- *To clarify core priorities and values.*
- *To highlight issues around the use and abuse of money in our culture.*

**21  SPIRITUAL PILGRIMAGE**                             (20–30 min, p. 94)
This lifeline drawing allows participants an opportunity to trace their spiritual journey and discover how it contributes to their well-being.
- *To raise consciousness about spiritual health as a component of well-being.*
- *To affirm life experiences that have shaped spiritual development.*

**22  SHOULDS, WANTS, WILLS**                                (15–20 min, p. 97)
A short planning exercise that invites participants to identify what they really
want to do about their health and what action they are willing to take.
  • *To separate the "ought to's" from the "I really want to's" in self-care.*
  • *To elicit commitment to one or two clear self-care goals.*

**23  WHAT DO YOU NEED?**                                    (10–15 min, p. 100)
This checklist helps participants identify qualities which may need personal
attention/development.
  • *To identify personal needs and values and determine ways to meet those
    needs.*

**24  REAL TO IDEAL**                                        (10–15 min, p. 104)
In this simple planning exercise, participants record their real and ideal health
status in a variety of life areas, then identify positive actions that could trans-
form the real into the ideal.
  • *To identify health ideals.*
  • *To outline necessary steps for reaching health goals.*

**25  PERSONAL PRESCRIPTION**                                (5–10 min, p. 110)
Participants write a personal prescription summarizing their self-care plan.
  • *To reinforce plans for positive health habit change.*
  • *To provide a reminder of self-care commitments.*

**26  MEET THE NEW ME**                                      (10–15 min, p. 112)
In this short closing ritual, participants imagine the health and vitality they will
possess one year later. Then they introduce themselves as if the planned
positive changes have already taken place.
  • *To publicly affirm personal goals.*
  • *To encourage each other and wish each other well for the future.*

**27  60-SECOND TENSION TAMERS**                             (1 min each, p. 115)
Five brief techniques for letting go of tension, including stretches, shakes,
deep breathing, and TLT.
  • *To relax body tension.*

**28  THE BIG MYTH**                                         (2 min, p. 117)
This stretching exercise asks participants to identify their "best" and then
discover that often their "best" can really be bettered.
  • *To challenge the myth, "I'm doing the best I can."*
  • *To observe that often we underestimate our limits.*

**29  BREATHING MEDITATION**                                 (1–2 min, p. 119)
This centering activity combines regular breathing with mental affirmations.
  • *To center attention and quiet thoughts.*
  • *To reinforce positive health images.*

**30  GRABWELL GROMMET**                                     (5 min, p. 121)
This humorous reading focuses on the "natural" consequences of negative
self-care habits.
  • *To poke fun at unhealthy patterns.*

© 1995 Whole Person Press 210 W Michigan Duluth MN 55802          (800) 247-6789

**31  GROUP BACKRUB**                                        (2–5 min, p. 123)
Everyone joins in on this gigantic, simultaneous backrub.
  • *To provide tension release.*
  • *To promote contact among participants.*

**32  MEGAPHONE**                                            (5–10 min, p. 125)
In this peppy exercise participants publicly acclaim their personal wellness
qualities.
  • *To affirm personal health-enhancing qualities.*

**33  NOONTIME ENERGIZERS**                                  (5–10 min, p. 127)
Participants tune into their whole person hungers and plan a revitalizing noon
break.
  • *To graphically demonstrate the opportunity for revitalization offered by the
    normal breaks built into the day.*
  • *To sensitize participants to the steady stream of needs they experience and
    to encourage them to respond creatively in ways that bring renewed vigor
    at the midday slump.*

**34  RED ROVER**                                            (5–15 min, p. 131)
Participants display their originality in moving across the room.
  • *To promote creative thinking and movement.*

**35  SINGALONG**                                            (2–5 min, p. 132)
Everyone joins in a musical break that reinforces a wellness concept.
  • *To raise group spirit and affirm a whole person wellness attitude.*

**36  SLOGANS AND BUMPER STICKERS**                          (10–15 min, p. 133)
Small groups invent slogans that could be used for posters or bumper stickers
in a wellness campaign.
  • *To reinforce wellness concepts and self-care strategies.*
  • *To spark creativity.*

## WELLNESS 2                                                    TABLE OF CONTENTS

© 1995 Whole Person Press 210 W Michigan Duluth MN 55802          (800) 247-6789

## 44  CARING APPRAISAL                          (45–60 min, p. 26)
In this whole health assessment, participants analyze the quality of their self-care habits (body, mind, spirit, relationships) as well as their other-care commitments (family, spouse, neighbors, creation).
- *To help assess self-care habits—body, mind, spirit, and relationships.*
- *To encourage participants to see that the "truly well" care for others too!*

## 45  SICKNESS BENEFITS                         (10–15 min, p. 35)
Participants use a seven-step process to track down the "benefits" they may gain from their sickness or its symptoms, then identify more responsible alternatives for getting their needs met.
- *To identify personal sickness patterns and their origin and explore the benefits of being sick.*
- *To promote personal responsibility for health.*

## 46  WHEEL OF HEALTH                           (60–90 min, p. 39)
This extended process helps participants explore the concept of wholeness by involving them in the building of a whole person model and examining the implications of their design. The process includes 3 parts: a) building the wheel model; b) exploring the implications of the wheel; c) self-examination.
- *To explore the interconnectedness between all aspects of health.*
- *To provide a model for understanding and describing wholeness.*
- *To stimulate the search for creative, nonlinear remedies that do not directly tackle the perceived problem.*

## 47  SELF-CARE LEARNING CONTRACT               (5–10 min, p. 49)
Using a concise goal-setting document designed for a multi-session wellness course, participants commit themselves to the course and assume responsibility for whatever changes they wish to make.
- *To secure a personal commitment for change.*
- *To activate personal responsibility for one's own health.*

## 48  WISH LIST                                 (5 min, p. 52)
This simple idea can be incorporated into the closure process for each content segment. Participants record all their dreams and hopes about how they could utilize what they have learned to improve their well-being.
- *To develop a written record of health-related desires.*
- *To facilitate the final goal-setting and planning process.*

## 49  ANNUAL PHYSICAL                           (30–45 min, p. 55)
Participants draw "real" body and "ideal" body portraits of themselves to highlight their physical assets and liabilities as well as to help them identify self-care goals.
- *To increase body awareness.*
- *To isolate areas needing more positive physical self-care.*

## 50  LUNCH DUETS                               (1–2 hrs, p. 58)
Participants pair up for a leisurely meal that accents the process of eating.
- *To heighten sensory awareness of eating.*
- *To explore personal eating patterns.*

- *To encourage increased self-care responsibility.*
- *To build skill in describing health problems accurately.*
- *To provide an easy-to-remember problem-solving tool for health concerns.*

## 58  WHAT NEXT?                                    (10–15 min, p. 97)

This simple process for ending a workshop day on a quiet note is particularly appropriate as a mid-workshop dismissal when additional sessions are scheduled for the following day.

- *To slow down the pace and encourage integration/application of the day's material.*

## 59  ROUNDUP REVISITED                            (1–2 min each, p. 98)

This quick closing exercise reviews the content and explores participants' satisfaction with the learning experience.

- *To compare original expectations with what was actually gained from the training event.*

## 60  CLEANING UP MY ACT                            (30–45 min, p. 99)

This activity is geared for participants who want to "clean up their act" by making several lifestyle adjustments at the same time.

- *To enhance personal vitality by increasing the frequency of positive health behaviors while decreasing the frequency of negative ones.*
- *To make incremental lifestyle adjustments one step at a time.*

## 61  ONE-A-DAY PLAN                                 (10–30 min, p. 106)

This creative process helps participants formulate a 30-day plan for reaching specific wellness goals.

- *To identify specific goals to be pursued and rewarded in the month ahead.*
- *To review and reinforce the concepts presented.*

## 62  VITAL SIGNS                                    (10–15 min, p. 109)

In this powerful closing exercise, participants affirm directly the signs of vitality which they have seen and appreciated in each of the other members of their small discussion group.

- *To experience the health-enhancing impact of being affirmed by others.*
- *To provide closure for discussion group members.*

## 63  BODY SCANNING                                  (2–3 min, p. 113)

This self-awareness interlude teaches participants a technique for attending to tension spots in the body.

- *To heighten awareness of physical tension spots in the body.*
- *To practice a simple technique for releasing accumulated tension.*

## 64  CHEERS!                                        (10–15 min, p. 115)

Small groups compete in a contest for the most creative wellness cheer.

- *To reinforce wellness concepts.*
- *To stimulate camaraderie, creativity, and humor.*

## 65  EXERCISES FOR THE SEDENTARY                    (3–5 min, p. 116)

This energizer provides a series of stretches that can be done while seated.

- *To relax.*

* *To practice options for stretching and relaxation that can be used during long periods of enforced sitting.*

## 66 FINGERTIP FACE MASSAGE                    (10–15 min, p. 118)
Everyone experiences the revitalizing power of touch in this soothing self-care break.
* *To experience relaxation and revitalization.*
* *To practice a simple self-care technique.*

## 67 GOOD MORNING WORLD                         (3–5 min, p. 121)
This sequence of gentle yoga stretches and rhythmic breathing is guaranteed to energize the group.
* *To get centered and activate mind/body energy.*
* *To increase oxygen supply and release muscle tension.*

## 68 I'M DEPRESSED!                              (2–5 min, p. 123)
This interlude demonstrates the mind/body connection and the absurdity of incongruent feelings and posture.
* *To illustrate the relationship between feelings and nonverbal expression.*
* *To discharge energy.*

## 69 TAKE A DEEP BREATH                          (10 min, p. 125)
This simple exercise teaches a five-minute relaxation routine that everyone knows and anyone can use.
* *To reduce body tension.*

## 70 UP, UP AND AWAY                             (2–5 min, p. 128)
In this uplifting exercise, participants learn the value of relaxed breathing.
* *To demonstrate proper breathing as a tension-reducing activity.*

## 71 WORKING COFFEE BREAK            (time varies with task, p. 130)
This novel approach to a simple time-tested technique teaches valuable self care lessons while providing a break in the action.
* *To revitalize body, mind, and spirit.*
* *To promote a high level of involvement among participants.*

## 72 YOU ASKED FOR IT                            (4–10 min, p. 132)
This high-energy exercise helps people practice asking directly for what they want.
* *To identify needs.*
* *To overcome the fear of asking for what you need.*

## WELLNESS 3                                           TABLE OF CONTENTS

**80  WELLNESS CULTURE TEST**                                    (60–90 min, p. 22)
Participants examine the influence of their environment on their personal
wellness habits by answering Ardell's tongue-in-cheek wellness culture test
and discussing the serious issues that it raises. They then take steps to
reshape their cultural norms in a health-enhancing direction.
  • *To illustrate the force that cultural norms exert over our lifestyle decisions.*
  • *To analyze assumptions about the proper and healthful way to live.*
  • *To facilitate the development of positive health-enhancing norms.*

**81  PATHOLOGY OF NORMALCY**                                    (5 min, p. 29)
This satirical reading highlights the absurdity of powerful cultural norms that
are antithetical to lifelong well-being.
  • *To recognize how cultural norms work against the wellness lifestyle.*

**82  WELL CARDS**                                               (30–45 min, p. 32)
Participants interpret wellness-oriented messages that they draw from a deck
of cards and examine the implications for creating healthier lifestyles.
  • *To assess current lifestyle habits based on a wide variety of wellness
    messages.*
  • *To expand positive wellness attitudes and behaviors.*

**83  HEALTH LIFELINES**                                         (75–90 min, p. 37)
In this multistage exercise, participants draw their health lifelines, examining
the patterns and critical incidents along the way. After writing autobiographical
statements and "telling their stories," participants project their lifelines of well-
being into the future.
  • *To explore and affirm personal uniqueness.*
  • *To outline a wellness history, identifying the critical incidents and lifelong
    health patterns that have shaped well-being.*
  • *To stimulate self-responsibility and "taking charge" of overall life direction
    and the quality of well-being.*

**84  STAND UP AND BE COUNTED**                                  (15–20 min, p. 44)
In this wellness habit quiz, participants graphically answer ten lifestyle ques-
tions with their feet—moving from one side of the room to the other to demon-
strate their responses.
  • *To assess personal wellness lifestyle habits.*
  • *To demonstrate that health is affected by many varied choices.*

**85  AUTO/BODY CHECKUP**                                        (15–20 min, p. 49)
This quick health assessment uses the metaphor of the automobile to com-
pare maintenance required for our cars with self-care required for well-being.
  • *To assess personal wellness style.*
  • *To promote positive attitudes toward self-care.*

**86  CHEMICAL INDEPENDENCE**                                    (25–35 min, p. 55)
In this exercise, participants examine the reasons for—and the results of—
alcohol use in our society, then personalize the issue by analyzing their own
use patterns.
  • *To raise consciousness about the patterns of alcohol use in this society.*
  • *To explore personal relationships with alcohol.*

© 1995 Whole Person Press 210 W Michigan Duluth MN 55802          (800) 247-6789

**87  CONSCIOUSNESS-RAISING DIET**                  (10–15 min, p. 60)
Participants use Dr. Christopher's memorable questions to raise their consciousness about attitudes toward eating.
* *To examine reasons for food choices and eating patterns.*
* *To incorporate healthy standards for determining what and when to eat.*

**88  COUNTDOWN TO RELAXATION**                     (5–10 min, p. 62)
In this quick and simple relaxation exercise, participants learn to deepen their relaxation response. This whole person approach is particularly involving since it combines physical relaxation with visual and auditory stimuli.
* *To demonstrate the effectiveness of using all three primary perceptual modalities (kinesthetic, visual, and auditory) in a self-regulation exercise.*
* *To learn a rapid, self-regulated method of deepening relaxation response.*

**89  FIT TO BE INTERVIEWED**                        (45 min, p. 65)
In this between-session activity, participants interview people who regularly engage in an appealing physical fitness activity. It is designed to motivate participants toward an active personal fitness plan.
* *To increase interest in beginning a personal fitness program.*
* *To gain firsthand information about a sport, physical activity, or exercise.*

**90  JOURNAL TO MUSIC**                             (60–90 min, p. 70)
This exercise enhances participants' sense of well-being by helping them clarify vague and elusive feelings, images, and personal goals. The process combines personal reflection and writing with listening to music.
* *To enhance feeling-level reaction to life experiences by journal writing.*
* *To encourage the use of music to bridge the gap between the language of physiology and the language of consciousness.*

**91  OPENNESS AND INTIMACY**                        (50–60 min, p. 76)
In this experiment with openness, participants assess their self-disclosure patterns and practice the art of personal sharing.
* *To encourage self-disclosure in personal relationships.*
* *To assess personal styles and patterns of openness.*
* *To practice the art of sharing oneself with others.*

**92  THAT'S THE SPIRIT!**                           (10–15 min, p. 82)
Participants use a simple checklist to assess their current spiritual self-care habits and then review a menu of spirit-related energizers for enhancing health.
* *To assess spiritual life patterns.*
* *To explore spiritual activities that enrich and rituals that refresh.*

**93  FOOTLOOSE AND FANCY FREE**                     (10–20 min, p. 86)
This fantasy invites participants to visualize a course for their lives unencumbered by possessions, responsibilities, and commitments.
* *To explore unrewarding patterns of living.*
* *To clarify personal values and goals that are of deepest importance.*
* *To visualize specific desired lifestyle adjustments.*

**94  POLAROID PERSPECTIVES**                              (30–50 min, p. 90)

In this unusual action metaphor, participants compare their personal development to a Polaroid snapshot, projecting into the future to imagine how the ever-
sharpening outline of their lives will develop.

- *To appreciate personal growth and development.*
- *To stimulate an attitude of self-responsibility.*

**95  CLOSING STATEMENTS**                                (10–30 min, p. 97)

In this reflective and integrative process, participants pull together insights
from the learning experience and assess its impact on them.

- *To provide closure for the learning experience.*
- *To reinforce discoveries, insights, and resolutions made during the session.*

**96  DAILY WELLNESS GRAPH**                              (20–30 min, p. 100)

Participants learn how to chart the daily ups and downs of their progress toward higher levels of wellness. (5 minutes daily for a month)

- *To heighten awareness of the change process.*
- *To provide feedback about wellness-oriented behaviors in several life
  dimensions.*

**97  FORTUNE COOKIES**                                   (15–20 min, p. 106)

In this upbeat session closer, participants invent wellness fortunes for one
another and exchange them in unusual "cookies."

- *To reinforce wellness concepts.*
- *To articulate desired goals and changes.*

**98  HEALTH REPORT CARD**                                (25–30 min, p. 109)

In this closing ritual, small groups of participants affirm one another's positive
health habits.

- *To reinforce positive health habits and attitudes.*

**99  50 EXCUSES FOR A CLOSED MIND**                      (5–15 min, p. 113)

This humorous list exposes the resistance to new ideas for what it is—
rationalization for keeping a closed mind.

- *To illustrate how excuses deaden creativity.*
- *To discover personal styles of resisting the new.*

**100  BREATHING ELEMENTS**                               (5 min, p. 116)

Participants draw strength and relaxation from imaging their connection with
the four basic elements: earth, air, fire, and water.

- *To focus attention on conscious breathing.*
- *To enhance relaxation by visualizing images of nature and the earth.*

**101  THE FEELINGS FACTORY**                             (2–3 min, p. 118)

This energy stretch break demonstrates how various physical activities can
generate a plethora of different feelings.

- *To energize the group.*
- *To demonstrate the close connection between actions and feelings.*

© 1995 Whole Person Press 210 W Michigan Duluth MN 55802        (800) 247-6789

**102  LIMERICKS**                                    (15–20 min, p. 120)
In small groups, participants compose witty ditties with a wellness theme.
  • *To stimulate creativity and humor.*
  • *To reinforce wellness concepts.*

**103  BALANCING ACT**                                (5–10 min, p. 123)
Participants pair up to demonstrate the dynamic process of maintaining a healthy balance.
  • *To experience the give and take required to maintain health.*
  • *To illustrate the concept and process of balance as a health goal.*

**104  OUTRAGEOUS EPISODES**                          (5–10 min, p. 124)
In this energizer, participants recall their most outrageous behavior and relish the playfulness and the risk-taking embodied in their activity.
  • *To highlight the role of risk-taking and playfulness in personal vitality.*

**105  SAY THE MAGIC WORD**                           (5–10 min, p. 126)
In this short, simple exercise, participants design their own vitality formula and capsulize it into a personal "magic word."
  • *To identify the personal energizers that frequently brighten one's day.*
  • *To devise a unique personal reminder that will help recall these surefire nourishers whenever they are needed.*

**106  STANDING OVATION**                             (3 min, p. 128)
This affirming energizer adds to the positive spirit of a seminar as participants periodically request and receive enthusiastic standing ovations.
  • *To ask for and receive affirmation.*
  • *To promote a high energy level and positive group spirit.*

**107  WAVES**                                        (5–10 min, p. 130)
In this relaxing interlude, participants take turns impersonating the undulating movement of seaweed being washed over by waves.
  • *To let go, relax, and feel the rhythm and support of other people.*

**108  WEATHER REPORT**                               (5–10 min per partner, p. 132)
In pairs, participants simulate meteorological phenomena as they exchange backrubs.
  • *To release muscular tension in neck, shoulders, and back.*
  • *To enhance relaxation through imagery.*

## WELLNESS 4                                                    TABLE OF CONTENTS

© 1995 Whole Person Press 210 W Michigan Duluth MN 55802          (800) 247-6789

- *To explore a variety of options for promoting whole person well-being.*
- *To promote creativity and humor.*

### 117  HEALTH AND LIFESTYLE                              (60–90 min, p. 33)

The film *Health and Lifestyle* provides the centerpiece for a mini-workshop on various wellness topics.

- *To explore lifestyle issues related to health and wellness.*
- *To identify personal habits that affect health and target specific lifestyle areas for change.*

### 118  WELLNESS PHILOSOPHY                               (20–30 min, p. 39)

In this exercise, each participant creates a personal credo of wellness and presents that vision to the group.

- *To examine the concept of wellness as set forth by pioneers in the field.*
- *To create a personal definition of wellness.*

### 119  SYMPHONY OF THE CELLS                             (20–30 min, p. 44)

In this two-part exercise, participants get a "cellular" view of the various physical and nonphysical body systems and explore how each system contributes to the overall harmony of the whole person.

- *To provide an imaginative and fun introduction to the "whole person" concept of well-being with physical and nonphysical body systems working together for total well-being.*

### 120  DECADES                                          (15–20 min, p. 49)

Participants review life experiences with illness and self-care habits in different periods of their life.

- *To review personal health history.*
- *To uncover self-care patterns.*

### 121  TAKE A WALK!                                     (45–60 min, p. 52)

This exercise gives new meaning to the term "active learning"—as participants take a twenty-minute walk and compare notes on their experiences.

- *To exercise for twenty minutes.*
- *To explore potential supports for beginning and continuing a walking program.*
- *To demonstrate the power of creativity to make exercise more appealing.*

### 122  CALORIE COUNTER'S PRAYER                         (10–15 min, p. 59)

This exercise combines humor and meaning by using the 23rd Psalm as a metaphor for weight loss. Participants write their own "Personal Psalm" for behavior change.

- *To add humor to a weighty subject as a motivator for behavior change.*

### 123  SELF-ESTEEM GRID                                 (45–50 min, p. 62)

In this assessment of a key component of health, participants affirm their extraordinary qualities, rank themselves on characteristics of high and low self-esteem, and make plans to boost their self-image.

- *To explore the role of self-esteem in whole person well-being.*
- *To assess self-esteem and affirm personal strengths.*
- *To identify priorities for self-improvement.*

**124  WELLNESS MEDITATION**                          (15 min, p. 68)
The cleansing breaths of this affirming visualization allow participants to find inner harmony and peace.
- *To practice a health-enhancing centering and relaxation experience.*
- *To reinforce the mind/body/spirit connection in well-being.*

**125  EXPANDING YOUR CIRCLES**                     (20–30 min, p. 71)
Participants explore preconceived notions about who belongs in their "inner circle" and experiment with attitude changes that can build a wider support system.
- *To demonstrate that our attitude, not the worth of other people, determines who we will exclude from our lives and who we will include.*
- *To encourage the development of a broader, more varied support network through attitude readjustment.*

**126  DEPTH FINDER**                               (30–45 min, p. 75)
Participants use a checklist to explore their values, then develop a graphic representation of their personal value systems.
- *To reinforce the importance of values as a source of life meaning and shapers of health choices.*
- *To clarify value system components and affirm significant values.*

**127  LET'S PLAY**                                 (40–45 min, p. 79)
Participants explore the health-enhancing benefits of play in this lighthearted look at a serious subject.
- *To examine personal play quotients and styles.*
- *To rediscover the importance of play in a healthy lifestyle.*
- *To uncover barriers to play.*

**128  JOB MOTIVATORS**                             (40–45 min, p. 85)
In this examination of needs and motivation, participants determine their personal priorities for job satisfaction and assess the degree to which their current life work fulfills their top-ranked needs.
- *To examine the multifaceted reasons for working.*
- *To assess the degree to which one's job fulfills major work-related needs.*

**129  INFORMATION IS NOT ENOUGH**                  (20–30 min, p. 93)
In this reflection process, participants explore their beliefs about a personal health problem and discover how they can turn information and good intentions into appropriate action.
- *To recognize the power of beliefs and perceptions as motivators or barriers to action.*
- *To promote health-enhancing behaviors and increase self-care follow through.*

**130  BEAT THE ODDS**                              (10–15 min, p. 97)
In this simple closing, participants remember key ideas, reflect on self-care strengths and weaknesses, and identify new behaviors and attitudes they plan to implement.
- *To reinforce key concepts and increase transfer of learning.*
- *To affirm self-care strengths and pinpoint areas for growth and change.*

© 1995 Whole Person Press 210 W Michigan Duluth MN 55802        (800) 247-6789

**131  DISCOVERIES**                                    (20–30 min, p. 100)
Throughout the learning experience and between sessions, participants capture their insights in a journal, then periodically translate these discoveries into concrete goals.
  • *To keep track of key ideas and personal discoveries during the learning experience.*
  • *To apply insights to life situations and develop a plan for implementing healthy changes.*

**132  GIFTS**                                          (5–15 min, p. 106)
In this closing ritual, participants "take the wraps off" and affirm the benefits gained from their study together.
  • *To provide group closure and give feedback to the trainer.*
  • *To reinforce learnings and affirm insights.*

**133  WORK OF ART**                                    (30 min, p. 108)
In this closing summary, participants create personal "pop art" sculptures symbolizing their enlightened understanding of wellness.
  • *To articulate insights gained and provide closure.*
  • *To use visual/tactile forms to express wellness.*

**134  WHISPER CIRCLE**                                 (10–15 min, p. 111)
In this affirming small group activity, participants are quietly showered with positive feedback.
  • *To promote group cohesiveness and provide closure.*
  • *To provide positive feedback for group members.*

**135  12 DAYS OF WELLNESS**                            (5 min, p. 113)
Participants join in a carol celebrating the joys of wellness.
  • *To reinforce wellness concepts.*
  • *To provide an energy break.*

**136  ALL EARS**                                       (5 min, p. 115)
Participants use different types of ear massage to energize themselves.
  • *To learn a simple self-care technique for stimulating body systems.*

**137  AS THE SEASONS TURN**                            (5 min, p. 116)
In this series of gentle yoga stretches, participants use images of nature to help them relax.
  • *To release tension through conscious breathing and movement.*
  • *To promote relaxation and centering through balancing and imagery.*

**138  CLAPDANCE**                                      (5–10 min, p. 118)
This peppy movement routine incorporates rhythm, cooperation, and interaction.
  • *To loosen up the group and get people together.*
  • *To provide an opportunity for playful interaction.*

**139  FIT AS A FIDDLE**                                (5 min, p. 121)
This lighthearted poem pokes fun at the self-righteousness of the wellness movement.
  • *To put wellness in perspective.*

**140  JOKE AROUND**                                          (5 min, p. 123)
Participants join in a hilarious interpersonal contact sport.
  • *To demonstrate the power of humor as a healthy mood-altering activity.*

**141  NEW SICK LEAVE POLICY**                               (5 min, p. 125)
This humorous reading spoofs the "blame the victim" attitude taken by some
sick leave policies.
  • *To provide an amusing look at a serious subject.*

**142  ON PURPOSE**                                          (10 min, p. 127)
Participants discover the power of purpose during this exercise in concentra-
tion and repetition.
  • *To explore the role of intentionality in healthy lifestyle choices.*

**143  SENSORY RELAXATION**                                  (5–10 min, p. 129)
Participants focus on sensory awareness in this suggestive relaxation routine.
  • *To reduce tension through the use of imagination and attention to sensa-
    tion.*

**144  TWENTY REASONS**                                      (5 min, p. 132)
Participants brainstorm motivations behind negative and positive self-care
habits.
  • *To generate ideas on a specific topic.*

© 1995 Whole Person Press 210 W Michigan Duluth MN 55802          (800) 247-6789

- *To explore self-care patterns.*
- *To get acquainted.*

**153  STATE FLAG**                                    (10–15 min, p. 37)
In this imaginative exercise, participants design a state flag that represents their current state of well-being.
- *To create a visual metaphor for personal wellness.*

**154  WORK APGAR**                                    (10–15 min, p. 40)
Participants measure their satisfaction with the function of their work systems using a quick, reliable scale, and then explore ways to increase their satisfaction levels on the job.
- *To explore satisfaction at work.*
- *To promote healthy work relationships.*

**155  VALUES AND SELF-CARE CHOICES**                  (20–30 min, p. 45)
Participants examine what constitutes a value and whether their self-care choices agree with their values.
- *To examine personal values and how they are translated into life choices.*
- *To realign values and act on them.*

**156  ASSERTIVE CONSUMER**                            (40–50 min, p. 49)
This exercise empowers individuals to express their health care needs assertively by writing a letter to people/organizations able to address their concerns.
- *To become proactive about personal health.*
- *To assert health care needs.*

**157  MEALTIME MEDITATION**                           (10–15 min, p. 56)
In this relaxing, sensory meditation, participants tune in to options for nurturing themselves at mealtime.
- *To relax before mealtime and recognize bodily signs of hunger*

**158  HEALTHY EXERCISE**                              (20–60 min, p. 61)
This short video and self-analysis process stimulates, inspires, and empowers participants to seek the health benefits of an exercise they can enjoy.
- *To learn about the effects of exercise on overall health, longevity, and risk factors for disease.*
- *To assess personal exercise patterns, confront barriers to regular exercise, and choose an enjoyable fitness activity.*

**159  IMAGERY FOR A HEALTHY HEART**                   (10–15 min, p. 63)
This directed daydream technique evens out blood pressure and helps maintain open arteries and a strong, healthy heart.
- *To practice visualization and sensory imaging techniques.*
- *To learn a practical technique for maintaining a healthy circulatory system.*

**160  SEVENTH INNING STRETCH**                        (5–10 min, p. 68)
In this invigorating exercise, participants combine fantasy with systematic relaxation skills to stretch each muscle group in the body.
- *To relax and revitalize the body and mind.*
- *To connect actions in a relaxation sequence with memorable imagery cues.*

© 1995 Whole Person Press 210 W Michigan Duluth MN 55802      (800) 247-6789

**161  MENTAL HEALTH INDEX**                        (30–45 min, p. 71)
Participants define mental health, learn about six common mental health problems, assess their own mental health, and discuss strategies for caring for themselves and others when problems occur.
  • *To promote mental health.*
  • *To increase awareness of common mental health problems, symptoms, and treatments.*
  • *To provide an introduction for EAP services.*

**162  SEVEN WAYS OF KNOWING**                      (60–90 min, p. 76)
Participants explore all seven of their intelligences with this creative, affirming tribute to differing gifts.
  • *To expand understanding of multimodal intelligence.*
  • *To identify personal strengths and problem-solving style.*
  • *To practice strategies for enhancing intelligences.*

**163  RELATIONSHIP REPORT CARD**                   (30–40 min, p. 85)
Participants examine the health of their primary relationships and friendships by completing a report card covering positive and negative characteristics for each relationship.
  • *To promote healthy relationships.*
  • *To reflect on which relationships to nurture, which to release, and where to build new relationships.*

**164  SPIRITUAL FINGERPRINT**                      (60 min, p. 89)
In this playful, right-brain exercise, participants create a work of art which symbolizes their current spirituality, then reflect upon ways to nourish their spirit.
  • *To explore personal spirituality from a new perspective.*
  • *To identify spiritual needs and ways to nurture them.*

**165  LEISURE PURSUITS**                           (20–30 min, p. 93)
In this expansive assessment and exploration of needs met by work and play, participants discover their priorities and possibilities for leisure pursuits.
  • *To evaluate the balance between work and leisure.*
  • *To identify needs met by work and leisure pursuits.*
  • *To explore affirmative activities for meeting leisure needs.*

**166  COMMERCIAL SUCCESS**                         (15–20 min, p. 97)
This exercise provides a creative way for participants to synthesize learning at the end of a session, working in teams to develop and perform a commercial to sell key ideas to the public.
  • *To summarize information and reinforce learning.*

**167  IF . . . THEN**                              (15–20 min, p. 99)
This quick and easy planner challenges participants to imagine the consequences of continuing or changing their present health-related behaviors.
  • *To review insights learned about wellness.*
  • *To apply learning by planning for positive behavioral changes.*

**168  JUST FOR TODAY**                                    (15–20 min, p. 102)
This memorable planning process based on the twelve steps challenges participants to make concrete commitments to change.
  • *To identify specific short-term goals to improve well-being.*
  • *To renew commitment to change.*

**169  SELF-CARE BOUQUET**                                 (20–30 min, p. 106)
In this unique process for planning and closure, participants create a metaphorical mixture of flower essences designed to heal their hearts, minds, and spirits.
  • *To integrate learning about wellness and identify and affirm self-care needs.*
  • *To provide closure.*

**170  TAKE THE PLEDGE**                                   (10–15 min, p. 110)
The power of a promise is apparent in this lighthearted closing pledge of allegiance to wellness goals.
  • *To make a commitment to personal health goals.*

**171  CHOOSE WELLNESS ANYWAY**                            (3–5 min, p. 113)
This lively exercise engages participants in a high-spirited litany asserting principles of wellness.
  • *To affirm a wellness way of life.*

**172  CLEANSING BREATH**                                  (3–5 min, p. 115)
Participants experiment with a yoga breathing technique that is a powerful natural tranquilizer.
  • *To quiet and balance the mind and emotions.*
  • *To promote relaxation.*

**173  FOR THE HEALTH OF IT**                              (5–10 min, p. 117)
Group members are invited to kick up their heels in a dance for fun and fitness.
  • *To enjoy the health benefits of dancing.*
  • *To stimulate interest in dance as a natural and fun way to exercise.*

**174  HEALTHY SINGALONG**                                 (3–5 min, p. 119)
Everyone will enjoy this playful, fun to sing ditty that celebrates good health.
  • *To laugh and play as a group.*

**175  LUDICROUS WORKSHOPS**                               (15–20 min, p. 121)
In this hilarious exercise, group members create outrageous courses for an absurd continuing education curriculum.
  • *To blow off steam and get energized through humor and laughter.*

**176  NIGHT SKY**                                         (8–10 min, p. 124)
In this awe-inspiring guided image, participants search the heavens for a sense of cosmic meaning and connectedness.
  • *To tap into creative energies and explore inner truths.*
  • *To engender a sense of connection to the cosmos.*

© 1995 Whole Person Press 210 W Michigan Duluth MN 55802          (800) 247-6789

**177  PERSONAL VITALITY KIT**                              (5 min, p. 127)
Everyone receives an envelope of symbolic reminders to stimulate whole person self-care.
   • *To reinforce self-care concepts and practices.*
   • *To encourage creativity and humor.*

**178  SIGHTS FOR SORE EYES**                        (1–2 min each, p. 129)
In this revitalizing self-care break, participants practice four techniques for relieving tension and strain in an often-neglected body part.
   • *To learn strategies for reducing eyestrain and tension.*
   • *To provide a relaxation break.*

**179  STIMULATE AND INTEGRATE**                         (4–5 min, p. 132)
This lively exercise provides motion which integrates both sides of the body while stimulating the mind.
   • *To become energized and mentally alert.*

**180  STRIKE THREE**                                      (3 min, p. 134)
This touching reading offers a childlike truth about healthy self-esteem.
   • *To stimulate positive self-esteem.*

# 8
# Contributors

The *Structured Exercises in Stress Management* and *Wellness Promotion* series are grounded in the philosophy of the Big Circle—experienced teachers and presenters sharing the best of their knowledge with others in the field, so that more people can be encouraged to develop and maintain healthy, satisfying lifestyles. The *Contributors* section highlights those seasoned veterans who have so generously shared their expertise in these volumes.

## CONTRIBUTORS

**Donald B Ardell**, PhD. Director, The Wellness Center—HRC/SHS, University of Central Florida, Orlando FL 32816-2453. ardell@pegasus.cc.ucf.edu (e-mail). 407/823-2453 (w) . Donald B Ardell wrote the landmark book *High Level Wellness: An Alternative to Doctors, Drugs, and Disease* and has since written twelve others, including *Die Healthy* and his latest, *The Meaning of Life: A Wellness View* (Whole Person Press, 1996). Since 1985, Don has produced 39 editions of the provocative and usually hilarious *Ardell Wellness Report.* (For a sample copy, send a SASE to Dr. Ardell.) *W3.80, W4.111, W5.171*

**Glenn Q Bannerman**. President of Bannerman Family Celebration Services, Inc, Box 399, Montreat NC 28757. 704/669-7323. Professor Emeritus of the Presbyterian School of Christian Education, Richmond VA. Glenn is a specialist in church recreation and outdoor education. He has conducted workshops throughout the US, as well as overseas in twelve foreign countries. His group experiences range from movement exercises and clog dancing to gaming, puppetry, crafts, and camping. He is coauthor of *Guide for Recreation Leaders,* and author of five LP American Mountain Music and Dance records. *S4.112, S4.138, W4.138*

**Kent D Beeler**, EdD. 6025 Compton Street, Indianapolis IN 46220-2003. 317/259-8064. Kent is a health psychologist and an active advocate of wellness at the college and university level. His experiential workshops have been popular with campus and professional groups interested in personal lifestyle promotion. Kent is a year-round, recreational runner. *S4.116, W3.75, W3.79, W3.82, W3.89*

**Martha Belknap**, MA. 1170 Dixon Road, Gold Hill, Boulder CO 80302. 303/447-9642. Marti is an educational consultant who specializes in creative relaxation and stress management skills. She has 30 years of teaching experience at all levels. Marti offers relaxation workshops and creativity courses through schools, universities, hospitals, and businesses. She is the author of *Taming Your Dragons,* and *Taming More Dragons,* two books and a cassette tape of creative relaxation activities for home and school. *S1.2, S2.68, S3.101, W1.23, W1.29, W2.67, W3.85, W3.100, W3.103, W4.137*

**Jan Berry-Schroeder**, MEd. 5676 N Pennsylvania, Indianapolis IN 46220. 317/255-1172. Jan is a consultant, therapist, musician, and writer. She specializes in bereavement, stress management, conflict resolution, women's issues, and self-esteem. She has extensive experience in Employee Assistance Programs and integrating wellness into the workplace. *S3.104*

**Thomas G Boman**, PhD. Professor, Dept of Education, University of Minnesota–Duluth, Duluth MN 55812. 218/726-7157 (w), 218/724-2317 (h). Tom is a practicing educator, in-service trainer, and program developer. His work with teachers at all levels of experience allows him ample opportunity to study the secrets of maintaining professional and personal vitality. Tom holds a PhD in Educational Psychology, MA in Curriculum and Instruction, BS in Chemistry. *S2.43, W1.8, W2.71*

**Richard Boyum**, EdD. Senior Psychologist, University of Wisconsin–Eau Claire, Eau Claire WI 54702. 715/836-5521 (w), 715/874-6222 (h). Dr Boyum has been a practicing psychologist, counselor, and teacher at UW–Eau Claire since 1973. His specialities include the use of guided imagery and metaphor in creating healthier behaviors. He also works with individuals, families, and organizations in creating behavioral changes through the use of both individual and systems models. *S4.125*

**Lucia Capacchione**, MA, PhD. PO Box 1355, Cambria CA 93428. 310/281-7495 (w), 805/546-1424 (h). Lucia is an art therapist, seminar leader, and corporate consultant. She is the author of nine books, including *The Creative Journal* (with versions for adults, teens and children), *The Well-Being Journal, Lighten Up Your Body, Lighten Up Your Life,* and *The Picture of Health.* After healing herself from a collagen disease through creative journaling, Lucia has dedicated her professional life to researching right brain approaches to healing and empowering individuals and organizations with new vision and innovative healing alternatives. Her best-known books, *The Power of Your Other Hand* and *Recovery of your Inner Child,* open new doors to self-health. *S4.119, W4.126*

**Linda Carrigan**. Manager, Product Development, Northwestern National Life Insurance, 20 Washington Ave South, Minneapolis MN 55401. 612/342-3717. Project developer for *The Stress Kit,* Linda received her BS in Community Health Education from the University of Wisconsin–La Crosse in 1979. Wellness is a way of life for Linda, both personally and professionally. *S1.5, W1.15*

**Jim Cathcart**, CSP, CPAE. PO Box 9075, La Jolla CA 92038. 619/558-8855. Jim is the author of *Relationship Selling* and *The Acorn Principle,* as well as an internationally-known speaker and past president of the National Speakers Association. *S3.97*

**Larry Chapman**, MPH. President, Corporate Health Designs, PO Box 55056, Seattle WA 98155. 206/364-3448. Larry is a consultant, trainer, and conference speaker. He has extensive experience in wellness programs in the workplace setting where he specializes in corporate health management, wellness programming, and designing benefit and incentive programs. *W4.126*

**Sandy Christian**, MSW. Editor, Product Development Team, Whole Person Associates, 210 W Michigan St, Duluth MN 55802. 218/727-0500 (w), 218/728-3916 (h). Editor of Volumes 5 of *Structured Exercises in Stress Management* and *Wellness Promotion,* Sandy is a licensed independent clinical social worker and a licensed marriage and family therapist. In her work as a therapist, teacher, trainer, and consultant, Sandy has maintained a lively whole person focus in health and stress management. *S2.54*

**Grant Christopher**, MD. MeritCare Clinic in Bemidji, 12333 4th St NW, Bemidji MN 56601. 218/751-1280 (w). Grant is a board-certified family physician who practices and promotes the philosophy of wellness personally and professionally in his medical practice and through the teaching of seminars on wellness. *W3.87, W4.124*

**Lyman Coleman**, MDiv, PhD. Serendipity House, Box 1012, Littleton CO 80160. 303/798-1313. Founder and director of Serendipity Workshops, Lyman has spent the past 30 years training over 150,000 church leaders of all denominations in small group processes. Author of scores of books, including a small group discussion version of the Bible, Lyman's innovative approach combines Bible study, group building, and values orientation with personal story telling. *S5.15, W4.109a, W5.146*

© 1995 Whole Person Press 210 W Michigan Duluth MN 55802      (800) 247-6789

**David G Danskin**, PhD. 180 Gray Mountain Drive, Sedona AZ 86336. 520/282-2372. David, a professor emeritus of Kansas State University, is the author of *Quicki-Mini Stress-Management Strategies for Work, Home, Leisure* and is coauthor with Dorothy V. Danskin of *Quicki-Mini Stress-Management Strategies for You, a Disabled Person.* He is also senior author of *Biofeedback: An Introduction and Guide.* David is now enjoying his retirement in Arizona. *S3.105*

**Dan Davidson**, DC. Director, Spinal Care and Wellness Center, 3531 Keagy Road, Salem VA 24153. 703/989-5477. Dan writes wellness songs including the four theme songs he composed as publicity chairman for the annual "Roanoke Valley: Alive and Well" wellness week. He is president of Alive and Well Music which provides wellness education through song. *W4.125*

**Robert C Fellows**, MTS. MindMatters Workshops, PO Box 16557, Minneapolis MN 55416. 612/925-4090. Bob is a widely-respected educator who combines his master's degree in theology from Harvard University with a background as a professional stage mentalist and illusionist. He regularly tours Australia, Canada, and the United States with his captivating presentations on self-responsibility in health. Fellows is the author of *Easily Fooled: New Insights and Techniques for Resisting Manipulation. S3.80*

**Emmajane S Finney**, MDiv. 224 W. Packer Ave, Bethlehem PA, 18015. 215/865-9777. Em is a Parish Minister in the United Church of Christ. She has special interests in Christian Education, women's spirituality, leadership of worship, and church-based community organization. *S4.139*

**David and Anne Frähm**. Health*Quarters*, 6873 Prince Dr, Colorado Springs CO 80918. 719/593–8694. Dave and Anne are authors of *A Cancer Battle Plan* (1992), *Healthy Habits* (1993), and *Reclaim Your Health* (1994). Besides writing books about health issues, they are codirectors of Health*Quarters*, a nonprofit health resource and information center and guest lodge. *S5.171*

**Joseph J Giacalone**. Program Director, Coors Life Directions Center, Regis University, 3333 Regis Blvd, Denver CO 80221. 303/457-4101. Joe is a health educator and manages a comprehensive health promotion program for students, faculty, and staff at a private liberal arts school and also teaches wellness to community college students. He has consulted with businesses and health care providers in developing survival strategies for dealing with the health implications of lifestyle and organizational change. *S3.75*

**Jerry Glashagel**, Consultant. 1714 N. Hudson, Chicago IL 60614. 312/649-9542. Jerry spent over 20 years with the YMCA in India, New York, Pasadena, Akron, and Chicago. He has degrees from the University of Illinois and Yale University, and enjoys facilitating groups, product design, writing, and training. He is currently a consultant in Russia, where he is helping small businesses develop. *S3.74*

**Joel Goodman**, EdD. Director, The HUMOR Project, 110 Spring Street, Saratoga Springs NY 12866. 518/587-8770. Joel is a popular speaker, consultant, and seminar leader who has presented to over 600,000 corporate managers, health care leaders, educators, and other helping professionals throughout the U.S. and abroad. Author of eight books, including *Laffirmations: 1001 Ways to Add Humor to Your Life and Work,* Joel publishes and *HUMOResources* mail order bookstore catalog and *Laughing Matters* magazine, and sponsors the annual international conference on "The Positive Power of Humor and Creativity." *S2.39, S3.107, S4.113, S4.134, S4.140, S5.177, W2.68, W3.99, W4.141*

**Lois B Hart**. President, Leadership Dynamics. 10951 Isabelle Road, Lafayette CO 80026-9209. 303/666-4046. Author of several excellent training manuals including *Connections: 125 Activities for Successful Workshops; Faultless Facilitation: A Resource Guide and Instruction Manual; 50 Activities to Develop Leaders; Training Methods that Work;* and *Learning from Conflict: A Conference and Workshop Planner's Manual,* Lois offers workshops, consultation, and presentations to all kinds of organizations who are interested in the development of their leaders and employees. *W2. 37a, W2.59, W5.145c*

**Tim Hatfield**, PhD. Counselor Education, Winona State University, Winona MN 55987. 507/457-5337. Tim is an educational psychologist whose teaching, public speaking, workshops, and consultation have focused on stress management, self-care, wellness, and lifespan human development. *S1.23, S124*

**Bill Hettler**, MD. President of Lifestyle Improvement Programs and Systems, 718 Linwood Avenue, Stevens Point WI 54481. 715/345-1735. Bill is a physician educator who has spent his professional life developing health promotion systems and materials. He is a cofounder of the National Wellness Institute. Bill was also the originator of the National Wellness Conference and has been an active contributor to both professional and popular publications. For the past ten years, he has been active in developing computer software to assist people in making positive health changes. *W3.84*

**Earl Hipp**. Human Resource Development Inc, 2938 Monterey Ave, Minneapolis MN 55416. 612/928-4936. Human Resource Development (HRD) offers keynote programs and training workshops that help employees gear up for the new world of work. Earl is the author of *Taming Invisible Tigers*, a dynamite stress management program for teens. *W3.81, W3.104*

**Donald Irwin**, PhD. Instructor, Des Moines Area Community College, Ankeny IA 50521. 515/964-6568. In addition to his teaching responsibilities, Don conducts numerous stress management workshops for audiences from housekeepers to University Regents' staff. Coauthor of the textbooks, *Psychology—The Search for Understanding* and *Developmental Psychology—Understanding One's Lifetime,* Don manages his own stress by practicing for the Iowa State Fair hog-calling contest, where he earned a blue ribbon three years in a row! *W4.143*

**David R Johnson**, MN, RN. St Francis College, 2701 Spring Street, Fort Wayne IN 46808. 219/434-3234 (w). David is an assistant professor of Nursing at St Francis College as well as an employee assistance specialist and certified marriage and family therapist with the Lindenview Counseling Center in Ft Wayne IN. He presents various community and corporate workshops whose topics include stress management, leadership, chemical dependency, self-esteem, grief, team building, and motivation. *W3.90*

**Krysta Eryn Kavenaugh**, MA, CSP. 955 Lake Drive, St. Paul MN 55120. 800/829-8437 (voice mail) 612/725-6763 (w). Krysta is a speaker, trainer, and consultant. Her mission is to take people "into the heart of wisdom." She speaks with style, substance, and spirit. She is also the managing editor of *Marriage* magazine. Her favorite keynote topic is "Romancing Yourself: Taking Care of You is Taking Care

© 1995 Whole Person Press 210 W Michigan Duluth MN 55802 (800) 247-6789

of Business." She also speaks on proactive support teams, turning adversity to our advantage, ecology, and customized business topics. *S1.4, S2.72, S4.144, S5.147, W1.2, W1.34, W2.41, W3.107, W4.123, W5.145b, W5.163*

**Merrill Kempfert**, MDiv. PO Box 2997, Corrales NM 87048. Merrill, a Lutheran clergyman, has been in the addictions treatment and health care field since 1972 in the Chicago and Albuquerque, New Mexico areas. He has served in a variety of positions which include chaplain, clinician, program manager, director of marketing, and chief executive officer. Recently completing his Master's degree in Human Resource Development, Merrill hopes he's closer to finding out what he wants to do when he grows up. *W2.54, W3.86*

**Julie Lusk**, MEd. Lewis-Gale Clinic, 1802 Braeburn Drive, Salem VA 24153. 540/772-3736. Julie is the editor of *30 Scripts for Relaxation, Imagery, and Inner Healing* (*Volumes 1* and *2*). She works as the director of the Health Management Center at Lewis-Gale Clinic and is the founder of the Alive and Well Coalition in Roanoke VA. She leads workshops worldwide on a variety of topics and develops wellness programs for businesses, colleges, and communities. Julie is a licensed professional counselor and has taught yoga since 1977. *S5.176, W4.135, W5.171*

**Jean Mershon**. Employee Development Specialist and Wellness Coordinator, St Louis County. Room 202, 100 N. 5th Ave W, Duluth MN 55802. 218/726-2446. Jean coordinates employee development and training for 2400 county employees. The wellness program offers a wide variety of health promotion programs and activities for county employees. *W3.96*

**Michael Metz**, PhD. Program in Human Sexuality, University of Minnesota Medical School, Suite 183, 1300 South 2nd Street, Minneapolis MN 55414. 612/625-1500. Originator of the *Play Workshop for Couples,* Mike has been researching the role of mature play in relationship intimacy for over a decade. Licensed Psychologist, Licensed Marriage and Family Therapist, and a Clinical Member of the AAMFT, Mike is currently coordinator of a marital and sexual therapy program. *W4.127*

**Pat Miller**. 1211 N Basswood Ave, Duluth MN 55811. 218/722-9361. In her consulting and teaching business, Pat Miller Training and Development, Pat leads workshops, conducts on-site team building sessions, facilitates retreats, and mediates conflict in the workplace. Her areas of expertise include communication skills, conflict resolution, team development, self-esteem, and stress management. *S3.73a S3.90, S4.122, S5.150, S5.178, W4.130*

**Jacki Mosier**, RN. Certified Family Nurse Practitioner. Acupressurist. 2018 N Crescent, Flagstaff AZ 86001. 602/774-8845. As a health care professional, Jacki has found a combination of traditional western medical practices, ancient practices involving energy flows, and spiritual recognition necessary to achieve good health and wellness. *S3.108*

**Belleruth Naparstek**, MA. 2460 Fairmonunt Blvd, Suite 320, Cleveland Heights OH, 44106. 216/791-0909. Author of *Staying Well with Guided Imagery,* Belleruth was trained as a clinical social worker at the University of Chicago, and has been a practicing psychotherapist for the past twenty-eight years. She is the creator of the *Health Journeys* audiotape series which grew out of her research and clinical practice with individuals who have life-threatening and debilitating diseases. *W5.159*

**Lyn Clark Pegg**, MS, LP, Doctoral Candidate in Human Resource Development. Lutheran Social Services of Minnesota–Duluth, 424 W Superior St, Duluth MN 55802. 218/726-4769. Lyn has lived the career development process. Twenty years and seven career decisions later, she found the color of her parachute at Lutheran Social Service. As a member of the management team and a psychologist at the Duluth office, she enjoys the best of all worlds—administration, counseling, professional consultation, and community education, all in the context of a Minnesotan culture that affirms and supports human services. *S4.131*

**John-Henry Pfifferling**, PhD. Director, Center for Professional Well-Being, 21 West Colony Place, Suite 150, Durham NC 27705. 919/489-9167. John-Henry is founder and director of the Center of Professional Well-Being. His PhD in Applied Medical Anthropology and post-doctoral training in Psychiatry and Internal Medicine uniquely qualify him as consultant to professional organizations concerned with preventing impairment. John-Henry specializes in coping skills training for professionals, particularly in medicine. *S1.13*

**Price Pritchett**, PhD. 13155 Noel Ct, Suite 1600, Dallas TX 75240. 214/789-7971. Price is the CEO of Pritchett & Associates Inc, a Dallas-based consulting firm specializing in organizational change. He has authored eleven books on individual and organizational effectiveness, including: *You²: A High Velocity Formula for Multiplying Your Personal Effectiveness in Quantum Leaps; New Work Habits for a Radically Changing World;* and *The Employee's Survival Guide to the Stress of Organizational Change. S5.180*

**Sandy Queen**. Director, LIFEWORKS Inc. PO Box 2668, Columbia MD 21045. 301/796-5310. Sandy is the founder and director of LIFEWORKS Inc, a training/counseling firm that specializes in helping people take a better look at their lives through humor, laughter, and play. She has developed many innovative programs in the areas of stress-reduction, humor, children's wellness, and self-esteem. *S1.26, S3.86, S4.118, W1.28, W2 45, W2.53, W3.74, W5.140*

**Ann Raber**, Director, Mennonite Mutual Aid Wellness Program, 1110 N Main Box 483, Goshen IN 46526. 219/533-9511. Mennonite Mutual Aid offers wellness programs for both adults and children. The sessions incorporate a Christian perspective, emphasizing the wholeness of the individual. The programs utilize active participation, small support groups, and local leadership. MMA also provides discussion guides for groups to study advanced directives, AIDS, Health Care Reform, and Medical Ethics. *W3.79*

**Ronda J Salge**, MA, RMT-BC. 5465 N. 650 E Churubus IN 46723. 219/693-9722 (h). As a music therapist, Ronda runs a private practice working with children. She has worked in acute adult psychiatric rehabilitation services, supervision of music therapy practicum experiences, and providing adult mentally retarded/developmentally disabled habilitation services. Ronda conducts workshops for community and professional groups on Journaling with Music and Relaxation Techniques. *W3.90*

**Louis M Savary**, PhD. 3404 Ellenwood Lane, Tampa FL 33618. 813/961-8046. Holder of doctorates in mathematics and spirituality, Louis is cofounder of the Institute for Consciousness and Music, and author of several books including *Sound Health* (with Steven Halpern) and *Passages: A Guide for Pilgrims of the Mind. S3.103*

© 1995 Whole Person Press 210 W Michigan Duluth MN 55802          (800) 247-6789

**Marcia A Schnorr**, RN EdD. Nursing Instructor, Kishwaukee College, Rt 38 and Malta Rd, Malta IL 60150. 815/825-2086 (w), 815/562-6823 (h). Marcia is the parish nurse of St. Paul Lutheran Church, Rochelle IL, 815/562-2744, coordinator of the Lutheran Church-Missouri Synod Parish Nurse Ministry, and an adjunct professor in parish nursing for Concordia University in Wisconsin. *S3.76, S3.84, W3.77*

**Keith W Sehnert**, MD. 4210 Fremont Avenue South, Minneapolis MN 55409. 612/920-0102 (w), 612/824-5134 (h). Keith is a family doctor who has become a leader in the medical self-care movement. He spends much energy in print (*How to Be Your Own Doctor—Sometimes, Stress/Unstress,* and *Selfcare/Wellcare*), and in person, urging people to improve their physical, mental, and spiritual well-being. He has an independent practice in St. Louis Park MN. *S3.91, W2.47, W2.57, W3.92*

**Janet Simons**, PhD. Permanent Adjunct Faculty member, University of Iowa School of Social Work–Des Moines Extension, 220 Avalon Rd, Des Moines IA, 50314. 515/222-1999. Jan, a psychologist in private practice with the Central Iowa Pyschological Services, has collaborated with Dr. Donald Irwin on the textbooks *Psychology—The Search for Understanding;* and *Developmental Psychology—Understanding One's Lifetime. W4.143*

**Gloria Singer**, ACSW. 43 Rivermoor Landing, 125 Main Street, New Market NH 03857-1640. 603/659-7530. Gloria's background as a social worker and educator are valuable assets in her position as Director of EAP Services, Resource Management Consultants in Salem NH. In that capacity she has enjoyed designing site-specific programs in stress management and wellness as well as training, counseling, and group work with employees and their families. *S1.3, S2.42, S4.121, W1.22*

**Mary O'Brien Sippel**, RN, MS. Licensed Psychologist, 22 East St. Andrews, Duluth MN 55803. 218/723-6130 (w), 218/724-5935 (h). Mary has spent over twenty-five years working in the field of community health and education. Her experience in teaching stress management, burnout prevention, and wellness promotion across the country has enabled her to be her own best caretaker as career woman, wife, and mother of two teenagers. Mary is currently a personal counselor and adjunct faculty member at the College of St. Scholastica, Duluth MN. She has ten publications to her credit, never tiring of sharing her enthusiasm for life, both on paper and in front of her audiences. *S1.20, S2.62, S3.100, S4.127, S5.159, W1.27, W2.63, W2.66, W5.160, W5.175, W5.179*

**John Sippola**, M.Div. 219 N 6th Ave East, Duluth MN 55805. 218-722-3381 (w). After fifteen years as director of Chaplaincy at Miller Dwan Hospital, John is currently tackling the challenges of whole person wellness in parish ministry. An innovative group leader and gifted teacher, John has specialized in mental health, drug and alcohol treatment programs, and recovery/relapse issues. *S5.164*

**Sondra Smalley**, MA. Licensed Psychologist. Clinical Faculty Member, University of Minnesota Medical School, 12701 Tealwood Place, Minneapolis MN 55356. 612/449-0525. Sondra is a full time organizational consultant in the areas of self-directed work teams and collaboration. *W4.134*

**Gabriel Smilkstein**, MD. Professor, University of California–Davis Department of Family Practice, Davis CA 95616. 916/759–2360 (w). Gabe has a long-standing interest in the family and the biopsychosocial model of health. Author of ten textbook chapters in family medicine and over fifty papers in peer review journals, his most recent studies relating to the influence of psychosocial risk factors on pregnancy outcome indicate the importance of social support. *S5.154*

**Ruth Strom-McCutcheon**, RN-CANP, M.S.N. Director of Nursing Operations, Duluth Clinic, 400 E Third St, Duluth MN 55805. 218/722-8364. Ruth is a nurse pratitioner specializing in women's health care whose work for over fifteen years counseling groups and individuals in the area of eating disorders led her back to graduate school in psych-mental health nursing. Ruth has recently traded the creative opportunities of providing health care services to college students for the challenge of assisting a thriving regional clinic to make a healthy transition to managed care. *S4.124, W2.69*

**Sally Strosahl**, MA. Marriage & Family Therapist, 116 S Westlawn, Aurora IL 60506. 708/897-9796. Sally has an MA in clinical psychology, trained at the Wholistic Health Center, and researched the relationship between stress and illness. In addition to her private practice in marriage and family therapy, Sally frequently presents workshops in the areas of stress and wellness management, burnout prevention, body image and size acceptance, and marriage enrichment. She particularly enjoys working with "systems" (family, work groups, agencies, business, churches) to help enhance each member's growth and well-being. *S1.8, S2.69, S3.89, W5.173*

**David X Swenson**, PhD. Assoc Professor of Management, College of St Scholastica, 1200 Kenwood Ave, Duluth MN 55811. 218/723-6476 (w), 218/525-3723 (h). A licensed consulting psychologist, Dave maintains a private practice in addition to his educational and therapeutic roles at the college. He provides consultation and training to human services, health, and law enforcement agencies and is the author of *Stress Management in the Criminal Justice System*. Dave also develops stress management software. *S1.18, S2.56, S5.153, S5.161, W1.16, W3.88, W5.175*

**Larry Tobin**, MA. Jade Mist Press, 1002 Maple Way, Stevenson WA 98648. 509/427-7082 Larry is a special educator, school psychologist, and national trainer on working with troubled children. He has authored *What Do You Do with a Child Like This?; 62 Ways to Create Change in the Lives of Troubled Children*; and *Time Well Spent*, a year-long stress management planner. *S4.142, W4.115, W4.136, W5.178, W5.179*

**John W Travis**, MD, MPH. 21489 Orr Springs Rd, Ukiah CA 95482. 707/937-2331. John is the founder of the first Wellness Center, author of *The Wellness Inventory*, and coauthor of *The Wellness Workbook; Small Changes You Can Use to Make a Big Difference; Wellness for Helping Professionals;* and *A Change of Heart: A Global Wellness Inventory*. His commitment is to providing safe spaces, conflict resolution skills, and the experiences of cooperation and partnership for helping professionals—replacing the authoritarian mindset of the illness-care industry and the culture at large. *W2.45, W4.118*

© 1995 Whole Person Press 210 W Michigan Duluth MN 55802          (800) 247-6789

**Donald A Tubesing,** MDiv, PhD. Designer of the *Making Healthy Choices, Managing Job Stress,* and *Manage It!* video series, editor of the *Structured Exercises in Stress Management and Wellness Promotion,* and author of the best-selling *Kicking Your Stress Habits,* Don has been a pioneer in the movement to reintegrate body, mind, and spirit in health care delivery. With his entrepreneurial spirit and background in ministry, psychology, and education, Don brings the whole person perspective to his writing, speaking, and consultation in business and industry, government agencies, health care, and human service systems.

**Nancy Loving Tubesing**, MEd, EdD. Product Development Director, Whole Person Associates, 210 West Michigan, Duluth MN 55802. 218/727-0500 (w). 218/724-7014 (h). With her roots and training in education, group counseling, creative problem solving, medicine, and theology, Nancy brings a truly whole person perspective to her teaching and writing. The soothing voice on most Whole Person relaxation tapes belongs to this author of *Seeking Your Healthy Balance* and senior editor of the *Structured Exercises in Stress Management* and *Wellness Promotion* series.

**Mark Warner**, EdD. Associate Professor of Health Sciences, James Madison University, Harrisonburg VA 22807. 703/568-3685. In addition to his teaching duties, Mark consults, writes, and presents on the topics of wellness promotion, leadership development, and organizational development.*S3.73a, S3.96, W3.76, W5.166*

**Randy R Weigel**, PhD. Associate Professor, Dept of Home Economics, University of Wyoming, Box 3354 University Station, Laramie WY 82071. 307/766-5124 (w). Through workshops, study guides, and media development, Randy specializes in making stress research understandable and usable by lay audiences. His training in human relations and education allows him to tailor programs to the needs of specific audiences. Randy has trained students, faculty, parents, ranchers, farmers, and helping professionals in stress management. *S2.47, S3.83, W2.70*

**Genie L Wessel**, RN, MS, FASHA. Administrative Specialist of Health Education, Frederick County Public Schools Health Services, 115 E Church St, Frederick MD 21701. 301/694-2156. Genie is now working to promote wellness in a large school system. She continues to share expertise in stress management and writing. She has been a founder and planner for the Maryland State Wellness Conference. *S2.64*

**Neil Young**, PhD. 728 14th Ave, Seattle WA 98122. 206/323-6310. Neil specializes in psychology and the arts, literature, and spirituality. As part of his concern for the wider world, he works regularly with Mother Theresa in Calcutta. He is currently developing a book on emphatic education. *W4.112, W4.142*